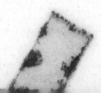

THE
SOUP-TO-DESSERT
HIGH-FIBER
COOKBOOK

THE
SOUP-TO-DESSERT
HIGH-FIBER
COOKBOOK

by Betty Wason

*How to add fiber and flavor to everything
you eat—appetizers, soups,
entrees, vegetables, snacks, lunchboxes,
salads, desserts . . . gifts from your
kitchen . . . great natural eating for
longer life and better taste*

Rawson Associates Publishers, Inc.
New York, N.Y.

Library of Congress Cataloging in Publication Data
Wason, Elizabeth, 1912-
The soup-to-dessert high fiber cookbook.
Includes index.
1. High-fiber diet. 2. Cookery. 3. Food—Fiber
content. I. Title.
RM237.6.W37   641.5′63   75-24234
ISBN 0-89256-001-0

Published simultaneously in Canada by
McCelland and Stewart, Ltd.
Manufactured in the United States of America
by The Book Press, Brattleboro, Vermont
First Edition

Acknowledgments

Among the many people who have been of help to me in collecting material for this book, I am particularly indebted to Dr. June Kelsay of the Carbohydrate Laboratory, Nutrition Institute, U.S. Department of Agriculture at Beltsville, Maryland. Not only was she generous with her time when I went to Beltsville for an interview, but she later clarified a number of points that had bothered me and sent me photocopies of useful articles on nutrition.

Ms. Ella Mae Stoneburner of the Seventh Day Adventist center in Tacoma Park, Maryland, was also extremely helpful, providing me with literature on the dietary and health background of the Adventists and suggesting useful Adventist vegetarian cookbooks. Through her, I was put in touch with Dr. Roland Phillips of Loma Linda University in California, chief of the epidemiological studies of the California Adventists.

I am indebted for information on the nutritional and fiber content of foods, as well as for recipes, to a number of food manufacturers, including Kellogg's, General Foods, Standard Brands, Nabisco, Quaker, Ralston, Pepperidge Farm, Roman Meal, and the General Nutrition Center, the latter a health-food chain with branches in forty-two states.

Articles in the two Washington, D.C., daily newspapers have furnished me with important background information: I must mention the outstanding job of consumer education that Marian Burros has been conducting in the food pages of the Washington *Post* as well as Goody Solomon's articles covering nutrition and diet in the Washington *Star*.

The charts in this book are based on a number of sources, from the Department of Agriculture's *Composition of Foods, Handbook No. 8*, the basic reference guide for everyone in the field, to the updated *Nutritive Value of American Foods in Common Units, USDA Handbook No. 456* (U.S. Government Printing Office, November, 1975), the Church and Church *Food Values of Portions Commonly Used* (J.B. Lippincott, 1975, 12th Ed.), *Nutrition in Health and Disease,* by Cooper, Barber, Mitchell, and Rynbergen (J.B. Lippincott, 1958, 13th Ed.), Frances Lappé's *Diet for a Small Planet* (Ballantine, 1975), and *The Barbara Kraus Guide to Fiber in Foods* (Signet, 1975). Special thanks are due to Birds Eye, Kellogg, Nabisco, and Quaker for supplying the fiber-content figures for their products.

The Barbara Kraus Guide to Fiber in Foods I recommend as a handy reference to supplement the charts in this book, because the author lists the fiber and calorie content of hundreds of foods that I did not have space for.

Many friends have been helpful, both in offering me use of some of their favorite recipes and also in doing some recipe-testing for me. To all of them I am more than grateful.

—BETTY WASON

Contents

CHAPTER 1

What the High-Fiber Talk Is All About

Diet and health are interrelated, as everyone knows. But now a growing number of medical researchers are convinced that *improper* diet is a major contributor to the ever-increasing menaces of heart disease and cancer (especially cancer of the colon), and to many other ailments and diseases as well.

It's not so much that specific foods are direct *causes* of these diseases (although some food additives are so blamed): primarily the harm lies in *what's been taken out.* By removing fiber, by making our carbohydrate foods too soft and refined, we have interfered with nature's efficient gastrointestinal system, clogging it up and throwing it out of gear. Not only does this help to bring about disorders of the bowel, colon, and rectum, it also appears to affect the entire circulatory system. Medical scientists now believe congestion in the gastrointestinal tract contributes to circulatory ailments such as atherosclerosis (hardening of the arteries), phlebitis, varicose veins, hernia, hemorrhoids, and gallstones. Some physicians also see this lack of fiber and related diet deficiencies as a factor in arthritis, diabetes, hypertension, strokes, kidney disease, even loss of hearing—and the list goes on. Lack of fiber is also seen as a *major cause of obesity.*

Dr. Burkitt's Discoveries

In 1970, Dr. Denis Burkitt, of Great Britain, a world-renowned cancer specialist, undertook a comprehensive study of the population in nine African nations. He was astonished to note that in all the areas he visited there were almost no recorded cases of coronary disease, cancer of the colon, the bowel disease known as diverticulosis, or of gallstones,

1

hemorrhoids, or appendicitis. *Nor did obesity appear to exist, even though the diet of the Africans he studied was heavy in starches and averaged about 3,500 calories a day.*

Why, he wondered, should these people living in quite primitive conditions not be afflicted with any of the "killer" diseases that take such an alarming toll of lives in the affluent Western countries, especially the United States and Britain? He concluded that the key factor must be environmental since *the diseases that dominate American and British mortality statistics are noninfective.* The death rate is due, he reasoned, to the way we live and the way we eat—and specifically he faulted overrefinement of carbohydrates, with white flour and white sugar heading the "enemies" list.

The African peoples Dr. Burkitt and his colleague, N. S. Painter, studied, eat very little meat and very little fat; their protein comes largely from vegetable sources—nuts, legumes, whole-grain cereals. But the carbohydrates they live on are all encased in fiber and most of them contain considerable amounts of moisture as well. None are concentrated, refined, or fiber-free. Therefore, Dr. Burkitt is convinced that fiber must be the essential ingredient missing in the Western diet.

Other Scientific Opinion, Pro and Con

Inevitably, there are critics of Dr. Burkitt's theories. Although chronic constipation is obviously related to insufficient dietary fiber, as are certain diseases of the bowel, many experts question whether lack of fiber can bring on circulatory diseases and malignancies. Others warn that too great an intake of fiber may result in the loss of important mineral elements: if wastes are carried off *too* soon, the body may not have time to absorb minerals into the bloodstream.

Some experts also criticize the overemphasis on wheat bran as the "missing ingredient," since *this is only one source of dietary fiber,* and one that may prove to be too rough a form of bulk for the systems of those with sensitive digestive tracts.

Dr. Burkitt contends that "you don't absorb cholesterol if you have a high-fiber diet," predicting that those who ingest sufficient fiber can "forget about fats." He points to a Dutch research project whose subjects, fed a diet heavy in oats and a leguminous grain, lowered their serum cholesterol levels significantly. His explanation: The dietary fiber in these grains triggered the excretion of bile acids which, in turn, help to lower blood cholesterol. But his critics consider this too sweeping a conclusion, and one that has been insufficiently tested.

Yet, despite controversies over details, the vast majority of researchers in the field view the high-fiber diet as beneficial. The question of dietary fiber will probably remain the focal point of nutrition research for a long time to come.

Sugar Shares the Blame

Equally as important as consuming more fiber is *decreasing* sugar intake. In fact, *many rate sugar as a greater menace to health.* The average *per capita* sugar consumption in the United States today is between 105 and 130 pounds per year, and approximately 60 percent of this is "hidden" in the processed foods we buy. When I first read that many brands of salt contained sugar, I couldn't believe it, but checking salt cartons in the supermarkets I found that *dextrose,* a sugar, was listed as an ingredient in nearly every one.

Here is a *partial* list of processed foods containing sugar: canned and frozen soups, *all* commercial salad dressings and salad dressing mixes, all gravy and sauce mixes, many of the "seasoned salt" and spice mixtures, mayonnaise, peanut butter, some frozen and many canned vegetables, prepared mustard, catsup, chili sauce, soy sauce, bouillon cubes, barbecue sauces, baked beans, hot dogs (both frankfurters and wieners), bologna, pastrami, virtually all commercial breads and other bakery products, many frozen ready-to-heat-and-eat entrees, such snack foods as wheat crackers, rye "toasts," cheese-flavored crackers, graham crackers, cheese spreads, all but two of the ready-to-eat breakfast cereals, shredded and Angel Flake coconut, and many so-called health foods.

This list does not include the obviously sweet foods: ice cream, cookies, cakes and cake mixes, pudding mixes, flavored gelatins, pancake mixes, whipped toppings, soda pop, most frozen and canned fruits and fruit juices (except those labeled "unsweetened" or "dietetic pack").

Why do American food manufacturers put sugar in products that have no need for sweetening? How do Europeans make superb breads without a trace of sugar or chemicals? And why add sugar to meat products, mustard, soups, and hot dogs? One can only suspect that sugar is added to cover up inferior products or to mask the taste of chemicals added primarily to prolong supermarket shelf-life.

An even greater scandal than sugar in bologna and soups is the large amount of sugar added to jars of baby foods. Analysis has shown that, in many baby foods, this proportion ranges between 27 and 44 percent of the total composition. Infants are "programmed" to want everything sweetened.

For years, dentists have warned that sugar causes tooth decay and mouth and gum disorders; now research links sugar to diabetes, acne, bronchitis, peptic ulcer, arthritis, even mental retardation, circulatory disorders, and heart failure. Not the least of its evils is its contribution to obesity.

Refined white flour and white sugar are equally useless nutritionally. The term "enriched," applied to white flour, should fool no one. In laboratory tests, of sixty-four rats fed nothing but bread made of "enriched" white flour over a period of ninety days, forty died of malnutrition, and those that survived were "severely stunted."

Proof of the Pudding

The effectiveness of a high-fiber, low-sugar diet has been dramatically demonstrated by a group in Santa Barbara who found it was possible to *reverse* atherosclerosis and other degenerative vascular diseases (including coronary insufficiency) by means of diet and controlled exercise alone. Given only whole-grain breads, no sugar, plenty of fresh vegetables and fruits, and small portions of lean meat (supplemented by chicken and fish), patients at Santa Barbara's Longevity Research Institute showed remarkable recovery. Within a thirty-day period, angina was reduced 100 percent in some patients, high blood pressure 75 percent, and diabetic patients experienced a return to normal coronary health without the use of any drugs whatsoever.

Another impressive report concerns the Seventh Day Adventists in California. In an eight-year study of 50,000

California Adventists, in which the causes of death among Adventists were compared with those of other Californians in the same age and sex groups, a striking pattern emerged. For every major cause of death, the Adventists' rate was significantly below the norm: deaths from strokes, coronary disease, and diabetes were 53-55 percent that of other Californians; digestive tract cancers, 65 percent, lung cancers, 20 percent, leukemia, 62 percent.

All Adventists observe the dietary principles established back in the late nineteenth century by their spiritual leader, Mrs. Ellen Gould. They avoid sugar and animal fats and eat large amounts of fresh fruits, vegetables, and whole-grain cereals. Approximately half of them are vegetarians, the others consume meat in limited amounts. They also abstain from tobacco, alcohol, coffee and other stimulants.

The first ready-to-eat whole-grain breakfast cereals were developed in the 1890s in Battle Creek, Michigan, an Adventist community, under Mrs. Gould's direction. At her suggestion, Dr. Harvey Kellogg, a surgeon at the local Health Reform Institute, and Charles William Post, an ulcer patient, created these early "health foods."

That dietary fiber, or "roughage" as it was then called, is important to good health has long been recognized. What is new is evidence that lack of fiber contributes to diseases that too often prove fatal.

Estimating Fiber Content

Despite the importance that health food enthusiasts attached to "roughage" in the early part of this century, for a long time many dieticians considered fiber relatively unimportant *nutritionally* because it was believed to be completely indigestible. But new research launched in the wake of Dr. Burkitt's discoveries has revealed that *total dietary fiber* is made up of several complex components and that each performs vital functions in the body.

Unfortunately at present the only figures available refer to *crude fiber,* the indigestible portion: authorities believe that studies now underway will show that some foods have three or four times as much *total* fiber as the earlier estimates indicated.

It's fairly easy to measure crude fiber: the application of certain acids to foods causes everything but the crude fiber to dissolve. But with this method the other fiber components are also destroyed. New methods for measuring all the elements which make up total dietary fiber have only recently been devised.

Even the crude fiber figures now available are *estimates only,* as Dr. June Kelsay emphasized when I interviewed her in the Carbohydrate Laboratory at Beltsville. In the same vegetable the fiber content will vary according to its age (or maturity) when harvested, the length of storage, and other factors.

How much dietary fiber do we *need* daily? No one can yet give a definitive answer. Very likely it will vary from one person to another, depending on already-established eating patterns and also on individual metabolism.

What the High-Fiber Diet Consists of

The high-fiber diet is keyed to these four principles:
• *Consume more whole-grain cereals and breads* and pass up or drastically cut down on white flour and other refined carbohydrates.
• *Reduce sugar consumption drastically.*
• *Choose fresh, frozen, or dried high-fiber vegetables and fruits.*
• *Cut down on both meats and fats.*
Another rule should be added. *Avoid synthetics and chemicals as much as possible,* especially artificially flavored and colored foods, those with "emulsifier added" or with "modified food starch." The term "emulsifier" in an ingredient list refers to sorbitan monostearate, a chemical that prevents bread from going stale, makes nondairy creamers dissolve readily, prevents stickiness in cake icings, and helps frozen products maintain stability through alternate thawing and refreezing during transportation and storage.

"Modified food starch" is used in baked goods, cake mixes, soups, pudding and pie fillings—and baby foods. Consumed in aggregate amounts, it can cause a swelling in the pouch of the large intestine. Many of these additives have been approved by the FDA because when each food was taken separately, the amount was considered low enough to be harmless; however, the long-range cumulative effect of ingesting many such foods could be very hazardous to health.

Note that it is primarily in convenience foods that one finds overrefined carbohydrates, "hidden" sugar, and potentially harmful chemicals. The best way to avoid them is to make more dishes at home from scratch—a practice that will also save you money.

Can One Lose Weight on a High-Fiber Diet?

What concerns many people is that the high-fiber diet seems to be the very antithesis of the popular high-protein/low-carbohydrate reducing diet theory. But in actuality, the high-fiber diet cuts out many carbohydrates—the *refined* "empty" carbohydrates that do us no good. Fiber not only helps to carry off wastes but also all *excess fats, sugars, and starches.* At the same time, foods high in fiber are correspondingly lower in *absorbable* starch and sugar and, because of their bulk, produce a sense of fullness, of *appetite satisfaction, which lasts from meal to meal.*

Can one lose weight on a high-fiber diet? Yes, very definitely, as we show in Chapter 3. But primarily it is a good-health diet, and if followed faithfully it will make you feel better, help to keep your appetite under control, and most important, help to strengthen your resistance to disease.

To me the beauty of the high-fiber diet is that it is taking us back to the kinds of foods nature intended man to eat. In other words, the high-fiber diet is a natural foods diet—it's that simple.

Making the High-Fiber Diet a "Way of Life"

Food is meant to be enjoyed; it should be one of life's greatest pleasures. Natural foods have more flavor than synthetics and overrefined pap. Bread made of whole-grain cereals has much more flavor than spongy white bread. Fresh vegetables cooked *au pointe* are delicious—when cooked properly, they do not need to be smothered in highly seasoned rich sauces. And simple fruit desserts make the perfect ending for a memorable meal.

The recipes in this book are intended to show how enjoyable high-fiber foods can be. After carefully studying charts to learn which foods have a high fiber content, I have developed hundreds of interesting, unusual, and mouth-watering recipes using them as the main ingredients. And because weight control is so important, I've included many recipes low in calories.

For me it was fun discovering that fibrous grains, seeds, and soybeans could become "conversation piece" ingredients, adding fascinatingly different flavors and crunchy textures to favorite recipes, and I was happy to discover that some of my favorite herbs contribute fiber as well as flavor.

Because I'm a down-to-earth person and know that most Americans will continue to buy their supplies in supermarkets, I have deliberately used supermarket products wherever possible. No diet is worth much unless it can be followed month after month, year after year, so that it becomes a way of life. The recipes and menu ideas in this book will, I hope, show how the high-fiber diet can become just that.

Teaching Children to Like High-Fiber Foods

The amount of soft foods and refined starches and sugars that children consume is appalling; it's not surprising that obesity has become almost as serious among young children and teen-agers as it is in the adult population.

Chapter 2 offers a variety of snacks, sandwiches, and drinks that will provide children with both good nutrition and plenty of fiber. Children who develop proper eating habits now hopefully will grow up with better teeth, fewer weight problems, healthier digestive tracts, and be better able to withstand disease.

A HIGH-FIBER DIET DICTIONARY

The following list defines and explains the terms used in this book, many of which may be unfamiliar. Brand names are used deliberately whenever I considered this to be less confusing, as for example, when a particular product is unique or differs in fiber or sugar content from others in its classification.

barley: a cereal grain used now mainly in the preparation of malt; *its fiber content is the lowest of all grains.*

bran: the outer husk of the wheat kernel. *Bran meal* is the crushed husk; it looks a little like sawdust but is high in protein, fiber, and is a good source of many valuable trace minerals including iodine. See also *whole-bran cereal.*

brown rice: the processed rice kernel from which the bran or husk has been removed but the grain has not been polished or refined.

brown sugar: crystallized white sugar that has been blended with 13 to 14 percent molasses.

buckwheat grains or groats: the kernel or seed of the buckwheat plant. Because this is different from the commercial Wolff's *Kasha,* also referred to as buckwheat groats. I call it *buckwheat grains* in this book. See *kasha.*

bulgur: cracked wheat, available in fine, medium, and coarse grinds. May be served (cooked) in place of rice, or as a porridge.

converted or parboiled rice: white rice treated before polishing so that nearly all the same minerals and proteins found in brown rice are retained.

cornmeal: crushed or ground field corn. *Whole ground cornmeal,* also called "stone ground" or "water ground," has far more fiber (2 percent) than the more common commercial "degermed" or refined cornmeal (0.7 percent). "Bolted" cornmeal is halfway between, with 1.2 percent fiber. See also *masa harina.*

crude fiber: indigestible plant cellulose in foods, also called "bulk fiber."

dextrose: one of the simplest (single) natural sugars present in foods; also called "glucose." Abundant in fruits and vegetables; extract of dextrose is used as a sweetener in many processed foods.

dietary fiber: the structural elements in plant foods which are largely but not completely indigestible. See following chapter.

fructose: also called "fruit sugar," it is found in many fruits and vegetables, usually in combination with dextrose. Honey, however, is almost pure fructose.

glucose: see *dextrose*.

honey: the natural syrup produced by bees; commercial honey has been extracted from the honeycomb and refined. Honeys differ greatly in flavor depending on the pollen in the flower or plant from which the bees gathered their food. *Raw honey* is less refined and thus contains more nutrients.

kasha: the Russian word for buckwheat; this is used commercially for Wolff's Kasha, actually *cracked* buckwheat groats.

legumes: all beans, peas, and lentils, whether the immature (green) pod or seed, such as in green peas, or the fully mature and dried pea or bean.

lentils: brown and yellow lentils are most commonly found in American markets, the tiny pink or red lentils in Oriental or East Indian shops. Needs no soaking and cooks more quickly than other dried legumes.

malt sugar: does not occur in nature but is manufactured from the starch in malt extract through enzyme action.

masa harina: literally "maize (corn) flour," this is cornmeal processed the Mexican way, the kernels first treated with lye, then ground.

millet: a cereal grain widely used in the Orient, Africa, and northern Europe; used mostly for animal feed in this country. There are many varieties of millet, but the *grains* referred to in this book are tiny yellow seeds; millet meal is the crushed grain with the husk, used primarily for porridge. Quite high in fiber content.

molasses: a by-product of sugarcane manufacture. *Light molasses,* the most delicate in flavor, has been more highly refined than the *dark* (also referred to as "medium"); least refined is *blackstrap molasses* which contains more minerals and vitamins but is disagreeable in flavor. See the chart, Nutritive Value of Sugars, page 237.

oats, oatmeal, rolled oats: as used in this book, these are all the same, the crushed kernel of the oat plant. "Quick-cooking" oats have been pressed finer than "regular oats" but have almost the same fiber and nutritive content. *Steel-cut oats,* available in health stores, have been cut very fine but retain full nutritive and fiber value.

pure bran meal: see *bran*.

raw sugar: the first crystallization of the sugar-refining process. It contains traces of minerals but not enough to make much difference.

rye flakes: the crushed or flattened whole-rye grain, useful in salads, breads, stuffings, and in breakfast "granolas": it can be eaten raw. Looks much like rolled oats.

soybeans: though a veritable "staff of life" in the Orient for many centuries, until recently this important legume was used mainly in this country for livestock feed. Now a number of food by-products are being processed from it, including Textured Vegetable Protein (TVP) used to make "meatless meats."* It is the highest in protein of all plant foods and one of the highest in fiber. *Raw soybeans* need presoaking and long cooking; *toasted soybeans* have become a popular ready-to-eat snack food. Some are sold as "perl-nuts" or "soy nuts." *Soy flakes* are raw soybeans pressed into flake form. They cannot be eaten raw but are useful in casseroles or stews. *Soy grits* are cracked dried soybeans; they are useful in breads, stews, or casseroles, but need considerable cooking.

sucrose: a double sugar found naturally in many vegetables, fruits, and plants; granulated and powdered white sugars are 100 percent sucrose in concentrated form.

sugar: as commonly used, the term means the refined crystallized product of sugarcane or sugar beets, but in scientific jargon, it means any of the several single or complex sugars that have been identified chemically.

---

*Some experts caution against too frequent use of TVP; in laboratory tests on animals it seems to cause kidney damage.

sunflower seeds: the whole sunflower seeds are useful chiefly for birdseed; it is the kernel inside the husk that is most palatable. *Raw* sunflower kernels are best for most uses; *salted* sunflower kernels, also sold as "sunflower nuts," are best for snacks.

triticale flakes: crushed from the whole triticale grain (a rye-wheat cross), can be added to cereals, breads, stuffings. Very high in protein and fiber, has all the virtues of whole wheat, can be eaten raw.

wheat germ: *milled wheat germ can only be purchased in health stores or pharmacies; Kretchmer Wheat Germ,* the product found in supermarkets, has been processed with honey and sugar and has less fiber content per weight. Milled wheat germ has less fiber than bran meal but is richer in minerals and vitamins.

whole-bran cereal: a generic term for all three of the commercial breakfast cereals highest in bran content: Kellogg's All-Bran and Bran Buds, and Nabisco's 100% Bran.

whole-wheat berries or grains: the whole grain which may be added "as is" to breads or other foods, but is usually crushed.

whole-wheat flakes: as used in this book, the crushed whole-wheat grain, which somewhat resembles rolled oats in appearance. Used generically, it may mean breakfast cereals in flake form, such as Wheaties.

CHAPTER 2

Easy Ways to Add Fiber

It's important to understand what is meant by fiber—*dietary fiber*. Fiber consists of the structural elements, the framework, of plant foods: husks, stems, string, seeds, skin, and also the cell walls that hold the softer portions together. In addition to plant cellulose, it also contains *pectin,* a powerful therapeutic agent which absorbs toxins and neutralizes harmful bacteria; *lignin,* a woody substance which adds bulk and absorbs moisture; and *hemicellulose* which triggers muscular action to keep wastes moving on schedule.

The completely indigestible *crude fiber* goes right through our systems, but some cellulose is broken down, releasing protein, complex carbohydrates (starches and sugars), and minerals and vitamins into the bloodstream.

Dietary fiber is found *only in plants;* there is none at all in meats, poultry, fish, dairy products, eggs, or fats. Its chief function is to rid the body of wastes, and it works like a miniature broom in the digestive tract, pushing down the wastes, absorbing juices to keep wastes soft, and liberating essential fatty acids—those that help to lower blood cholesterol. When there isn't enough fiber to do the job properly, it's as if a drain sewer were backing up with litter and garbage. Not only do harmful bacteria thrive in the "garbage," the entire circulatory system is affected.

Since it has not been determined how much fiber we need —and our individual needs vary considerably—a simple guideline is to consume enough fiber to produce easy, effortless elimination (or "evacuation," as doctors now term it) once a day, but no more than that. It *is* possible to consume too much fiber!

"Guesstimates" of fiber need have ranged from 6 grams daily up to 10 or 15 grams (Dr. Burkitt) or even 24 grams

(Dr. Reuben). But Reuben concedes that for some a third of this amount may be sufficient.

Cereal grains are major sources of dietary fiber but some contain far more fiber than others. Wheat bran and buckwheat lead the list; triticale (a cross between rye and wheat), rye, soy, oats, and millet all are excellent sources. But neither rice, barley, nor cornmeal rates well. Barley has less fiber than fresh peaches; 100 grams of brown rice has about the same amount of fiber as a half cup of fresh mushrooms. Commercial corn muffin mix has no more than biscuit mix: 0.1 percent.

Seeds, legumes, and nuts are excellent sources, but nuts should be eaten sparingly because of their high fat content. All vegetables contain some dietary fiber; certain ones are outstandingly good sources. It is possible to obtain as much fiber from two portions of high-fiber vegetables at dinner as from a bowl of whole-bran cereal at breakfast. One-half cup of blackberries has *more* fiber than one-half cup of Kellogg's All-Bran cereal. (See Vegetable and Fruit Charts, at the back of the book, pages 231–234.)

Good first steps for adapting to a high-fiber diet include the following: (1) Buy only whole-wheat and other whole-grain bread and cereal products, no white bread at all; (2) read labels on processed foods and avoid those made with refined starches and needless amounts of sugar; (3) get acquainted with products in health stores.

I have found health stores to be an excellent source of many high-fiber ingredients and sugarless snack foods not available elsewhere. Stores that sell whole-grain products in barrels or bulk make considerable savings possible, too.

For example, in the Woodlawn Pharmacy and Health Store, in my neighborhood in Arlington, Virginia, rolled oats were available in an open bin for 29 cents a pound when a 16-ounce (1 pound) package of Quaker Oats in the supermarket was selling for 59 cents. (If a store sells these flours and grains in bulk, you can buy as little as a dime's worth to try them out for flavor.) I used less than 55 cents worth of buckwheat grains in developing recipes for this book. These little grains have a nutty, almost sweet taste and, according to the USDA Composition of Foods chart, even more crude fiber than wheat brain. They can be eaten raw.

A number of high-fiber products formerly found only in health stores are now on supermarket shelves, particularly toasted soybeans and sunflower kernels, whole-wheat flour, rye flour, and unbleached white flour.

How to Read Labels

By federal law, *every* processed food must contain somewhere on its label a list of ingredients, and the ingredients must be given in order of content. When sugar appears as the second ingredient listed, you can be sure the sugar content is very, very high.

When the list includes "enriched wheat flour," it means refined white flour with some, not all, vitamins and minerals put back in. Unless the label specifies *whole wheat,* the terms "enriched" and "wheat" are deceptive.

It is especially important to read labels on breakfast cereals. Out of the 150 or more brands distributed nationwide in supermarkets, only *two* ready-to-eat breakfast cereals are free of added sugar or other sweeteners: Shredded Wheat, both large and spoon-size biscuits, and Grape-Nuts. The latter, though, is not a high-fiber food because it is made largely of toasted barley grains.

In addition to sugar (brown and white), note whether the ingredient list includes dextrose, corn syrup, malt, honey, or molasses, because *all these are sugars.* White sugar is the worst, because 90 percent of the cane or beet has been removed, leaving a residue of pure crystallized sucrose, nothing else. Brown sugar is only slightly better, and honey may be more harmful than white sugar, according to Dr. June Kelsay, medical researcher at the USDA Carbohydrate Laboratory. Dr. Kelsay told me that laboratory tests on animals showed that fructose, the main component in honey, synthesized even more fat than sucrose—which means that people who consume quantities of honey will tend to put on even more fat. Molasses is the only sweetener with enough mineral content to be of some nutritional benefit.

Sneaking in Fiber Here and There

Certain grains, seeds, nuts, and cereals are particularly useful in the kitchen. I keep a selection handy in glass jars so that on impulse I can sprinkle a little here and there in salads, casseroles, sandwich fillings, whatever.

Here is how they stack up fiber-wise (figures are based on 100-gram portions).

Wheat products

pure bran meal	9.1%
whole-bran breakfast cereal	7.8
40% Bran Flakes	3.6
crude wheat germ	2.5
Kretchmer wheat germ	1.7
whole-wheat berries, grains, or flakes	2.3
Shredded Wheat biscuits (no sugar)	2.3
Wheat Chex	1.6

Other grains

buckwheat grains or groats	9.9
Wolff's Kasha	2.0
millet grains	3.2
rye flakes (whole grain)	2.0
rolled oats	1.2
soy flakes	4.9
soy grits	3.0
toasted soybeans	2.8

Nuts and seeds

sunflower kernels (or nuts)	3.8%
peanuts	2.4–2.7
almonds	2.6
English walnuts	2.1
pecans	2.3
coconut (fresh)	4.0
coconut dried (sweetened or unsweetened)	3.9
pine nuts	1.1

(Dr. Burkitt gives bran meal a 9 to 12 percent fiber content.)

To demonstrate how a little fiber here and there can add up by the end of a day to more than 15 grams, I devised a day's skeleton menu as an example.

Breakfast:

1	medium orange, peeled, sliced	0.8 grams fiber	
1	large Shredded Wheat biscuit	2.0	
	mixed with ½ tablespoon		
	buckwheat	1.3	
	and ¼ cup 40% Bran Flakes	0.37	
	and 1 tablespoon dried		
	currants	0.2	
2	slices whole-wheat toast	0.75	
	with blackberry jam	0.3	
	(*not* seeded)		
		5.72	5.72

Lunch:

½	avocado	1.8 grams fiber	
	on ¾ cup shredded romaine	0.3	
	filled with ½ cup cottage		
	cheese	0.0	
	mixed with sunflower kernels	0.25	
1	slice whole-wheat bread	0.5	
1	apple (not peeled)	1.4	
		4.25	4.25

Snacks:

¼	green pepper, slivered	0.35	
1	small carrot, in sticks	0.7	
1	ounce toasted soybeans	0.35	
3	Swedish rye wafers or Triscuits	0.3	
		1.70	1.70

Dinner:

1	small broiled steak	0.0
½	cup green peas	1.6
1	medium potato, baked	0.6
1	bran muffin	0.7

1 raw peach	0.6	
mixed with ¼ cup chopped		
dates	0.6	
and 1 tablespoon dried		
coconut	0.2	
	4.3	4.30

Day's Total: 15.97

At Breakfast

EGGS

• *Scrambled eggs* can be fiber-enriched with: chunks of avocado, whole-bran cereal, pure bran meal, sunflower kernels, chopped parsley, chopped green peppers, chopped peanuts, or a sprinkling of buckwheat grains.

• *Baked eggs.* Preheat oven to 400° (hot). Place a dab of butter and a handful of Wheat Chex in each ramekin (one to a serving); put in oven until butter melts, then remove, stir Wheat Chex to coat with butter. Break an egg over Wheat Chex, sprinkle lightly with salt, add 1 tablespoon of milk to each. Return to oven until eggs are set, yolks still soft. Allow 5 minutes for 1 egg to a ramekin, 10 minutes for 2.

• *Poached eggs.* Serve over toasted whole-wheat bread or bran muffins.

• *Hearty breakfast nog.* For each serving, drop into blender 1 egg, 1 cup of milk, 2 tablespoons of whole-bran cereal, ½ teaspoon of vanilla—*no sugar.* Beat until smooth. This is a great liquid breakfast for those in too much of a hurry to sit down. Add a bacon sandwich (between whole-wheat toast) and an apple to be eaten en route.

MUFFINS

• Make up a batch of Refrigerator Bran Muffin batter (recipe on page 49) from which you spoon out as much as you need daily, then bake in a flash.

• Or make up a big batch of bran muffins ahead, bake and freeze in meal-size portions, to reheat as needed.

• Besides the muffin variations in Chapter 4, you may add fiber to commercial mixes by stirring in pure bran meal, chopped nuts, or chopped dried fruit.

Toast and Jam

• Whether you bake your own or buy, be sure to use whole-grain bread to make breakfast toast.

• Blackberry, raspberry, currant, and gooseberry jams all are fibrous if made with *the whole fruit,* not strained. All fiber has been strained out of jellies, however. Orange marmalade also has fiber (orange peel).

• Try this easy *Peach Nut Conserve:* To 1 cup of peach jam, stir in ¼ cup of chopped sunflower kernels (or toasted almonds) and 1 tablespoon of whole-bran cereal.

Pancakes and Waffles

• Of commercial pancake mixes in supermarket distribution, Aunt Jemima's "original" and the buckwheat and whole-wheat mixes stand out above the others for fiber content. The buckwheat doesn't even contain sugar, hallelujah! Other buckwheat and whole-wheat pancake mixes, as well as blends containing soy flour, can be found in health stores.

• Blueberries, chopped apple, coconut, nuts, seeds, and whole grains (including my favorite, buckwheat) can be added to any pancake or waffle batter.

Coffee Cake

• If you use a mix or a standard recipe with white flour, be sure to add bran meal to it, 2 teaspoons to a cup. Also add chopped dried fruits, apple, or nuts.

• This *Bran Topping* makes a quick streusel: Combine 4 tablespoons of margarine or butter, ½ cup of whole-bran cereal, ½ cup of shredded dried coconut, ½ teaspoon of cinnamon, and 1 tablespoon of brown sugar. Mix until crumbly, and sprinkle over top of dough before baking.

At Lunch

LUNCHBOX SUGGESTIONS

- Make all sandwiches with whole-grain breads.
- Almost any sandwich filling is improved by adding chopped sunflower kernels, especially tuna, egg salad, ham salad, or cheese mixtures.
- Date butter is delicious between whole-wheat or any dark health bread. Or add chopped dates to cream or Neufchâtel cheese.
- If your youngsters insist on peanut butter and jelly, substitute blackberry or red raspberry jam for jelly.
- Here's a high-fiber ham salad mixture: chopped ham, whole-bran cereal, chopped sliced radishes, raisins, and enough cottage cheese to hold it together (no mayonnaise).
- Best lunchbox fruits: pears, apples, banana, prunes, or fresh blue plums, dried apricots, and other dried fruits.
- Chapters 12 and 14 both offer recipes for cookies made at home with whole-grain flours and reduced amounts of sugar.

RESTAURANT LUNCHES

- When you order a hamburger, skip the bun and french fries; ask for coleslaw or salad instead. A *little* catsup won't hurt, but remember it is *high* in sugar.
- Avoid pastas, rice, or french fries; choose vegetables such as green beans, peas, carrots, or broccoli.
- If salad is on the menu, avoid high-calorie dressings; ask for oil and vinegar to dress your own, and use moderate amounts.
- For dessert, order fresh fruit.
- While waiting for your entree, fill up on salad or whole-wheat bread—not white bread and butter.

LUNCH AT HOME

• Enhance low-fat cottage cheese with two or more of the following: toasted soybeans, sunflower kernels, buckwheat grains, chopped green peppers, rye flakes, wheat germ, whole-bran cereal, chopped unpeeled apple or pear, currants, dried apricots, caraway, fennel, or sesame seeds (toasted), chopped parsley, chopped fresh coriander, or watercress.

• Other lunch salad suggestions: to green beans vinaigrette, add toasted sesame seeds and sunflower kernels. Make a "cooked salad" with leftover vegetables, top with chopped nuts. Add shredded carrots and/or chopped peanuts to coleslaw.

At Dinner or Full-Course Luncheons

BEFORE-DINNER APPETIZERS

• Raw vegetable relishes as well as olives (both green and black) boost your fiber intake.

• For dips, use yogurt blended with coarsely chopped nuts and parsley, or Humus (recipe on page 72), a chickpea dip.

• Make your own melba toast with thin-sliced home-baked whole-wheat or other health bread: cut into squares and slow-bake in oven until crisp and dry.

• With drinks, munch on toasted soybeans or salted sunflower "nuts" instead of potato chips.

SALADS

• Serve salads as a first course in the California manner.

• Add toasted soybeans, sunflower seeds, or uncooked buckwheat grains to almost any tossed salad. (Rye flakes are good, too.)

• For salad croutons, use Wheat Chex seasoned, if you wish, with garlic or other seasoned salt.

The Main Course

• For breading meat, poultry, or chicken, use crushed Shredded Wheat, 40% Bran or whole-bran cereals, or crushed Triscuits (these contain salt and oil).

• Thicken gravies and sauces with whole-wheat or soy flour.

• If you use canned gravy, add 1 tablespoon of bran meal first softened in ¼ cup of water, with chopped parsley and a little white wine.

• Thicken stews with whole-bran cereal or bran meal first softened with liquids; then cook at least 15 minutes after bran is added to blend completely.

• For bread stuffings in meat or poultry, use whole-wheat or other whole-grain breads rather than commercial stuffing mix.

• Top casseroles with a mixture of crushed Shredded Wheat, bran meal, grated cheese, salt, and pepper.

Vegetables and Side Dishes

• A baked potato is only slightly higher in calories than a serving of green peas, lower than limas, and if you eat the skin, you get extra roughage.

• Study the Vegetable Chart on page 231 to learn the fiber content of all vegetables and Chapter 10 for easy and unusual recipes.

• Instead of rice, serve cooked millet or bulgur (or the two mixed together) for more fiber.

• Increase fiber in white or brown rice with caraway seeds or crushed cardamom, toasted soybeans, buckwheat grains or groats added to cooked rice.

Desserts

• Fresh raw fruit is the best dessert.

• Instead of cakes or puddings made with mixes, make bread pudding using whole-wheat or oatmeal bread, also fruit cobblers, or crisps to which bran is added.

• *Yogurt desserts* are versatile, and yogurt is lower in fat than sour or sweet cream or ice cream. The culture that causes it to solidify also serves as a kind of antibiotic in the alimentary canal. But choose yogurt containing only the culture, not those thickened with vegetable gum and gelatin and avoid the sweetened yogurts. All the following combinations are interesting; add "according to taste," exact measurements are not important.

—Shredded coconut and a bit of whole-bran cereal.

—Blackberry jam or drained canned blackberries.

—Gooseberry jam, sunflower kernels, chopped apple.

—A bit of molasses, wheat germ and/or buckwheat, dash of cinnamon. (Use this mixture to top fruit or Carrot Cake.)

—Chopped unpeeled pears, a little pure maple syrup, crushed Wheat Chex.

• In making cheesecake, use yogurt in place of cream in the recipe, and finely crushed whole-bran cereal or Shredded Wheat in place of crushed zwiebach or other crumbs.

Bedtime Snacks

It is unwise and fattening to eat filling or rich foods at bedtime. You won't burn up calories (as you do after breakfast and lunch), and it puts your digestive tract to work, which could interfere with sleep.

The best snack is *fresh fruit*. Next best—ready-to-eat whole-grain sugarless cereal topped with fruit and milk.

A glass of milk helps some people to sleep. One of the nogs in Chapter 12 may fill the bill, or try a cup of hot carob "cocoa."

CHAPTER 3

How to Lose Weight on a High-Fiber Diet

During the first weeks that I tested recipes for this book, my weight shot up and I thought, "Who's going to accept a diet that makes you *put on* weight?" But a month later, when my weight was back to normal again, I began to notice that I no longer felt that urge to nibble between meals or to reach for seconds at the table.

Six weeks later, when I had stopped trying to lose weight, to my amazement I saw that the needle on my bathroom scales had dropped down and I even had to take in the waistline on pants and skirts more than an inch. I was eating more bread and cereal grains, consuming more calories, yet slimming down in the process!

Looking back, I realized that I had put on weight initially because I was testing dozens of breads, cookies, and pastries, foods I normally don't touch. When I finished that phase, it was not at all difficult to take off the few extra pounds I'd gained. I simply reverted to my normal diet—with one exception. I had learned to *like* such fibrous foods as buckwheat grains, rye flakes, soybeans, and sunflower kernels, and was slipping them into everything by choice.

This proved to me the truth of claims made by the proponents of the high-fiber diet: (1) high-fiber foods not only satisfy hunger quickly but also *keep one feeling satisfied* from meal to meal, and (2) one can actually eat more and gain less, because dietary fiber quickly rids the digestive tract of excess starches, sugars, and fats. That is, providing *refined* starches, sugars, and excess fats are also avoided.

Special Rules for Weight-Watchers

• *Don't skimp on breakfast.* This is the time to get the biggest portion of your day's fiber. Every morning have whole-grain breakfast cereal or whole-grain bread, or both, plus fresh fruit (not juices).

• *Eat as much as you like* of vegetables that are low in calories but high in fiber.

• *Take only modest portions* of high-calorie vegetables such as corn, white and sweet potatoes, green peas, limas, *all* legumes. All are good fiber sources; don't pass them up, just limit the amount.

• *Eat chicken and fish in preference to meat* (even lean meat).

• *No sweets or desserts, no refined carbohydrate snacks.*

• *Skip dinner entirely every now and then;* satisfy the urge to eat by chewing on raw vegetables and/or raw fruits.

• *Get exercise every day.* (Choose whichever suits your schedule best: a gym workout, jogging, daily push-ups, long walks, any favorite active sport—as long as you do *something* to burn up calories.)

• *Don't count calories.* Instead, consider the *kinds of calories* you are eating. Are they furnished largely by fats, refined starches, or sugar? If so, discontinue them. Or are they mainly unrefined carbohydrates, proteins, and the natural sugar of vegetables and fruits? If any of the latter three, enjoy them—in reasonable portions, of course. Naturally, the less you consume overall, the faster pounds will melt away.

• *Cut down drastically on both alcohol and carbonated drinks.* Alcohol is another form of sugar and thus contains "empty calories."

The Sugar Syndrome

Just cutting out sugar from your diet will cause you to lose weight—but, remember, this means avoiding processed foods with "hidden" sugar as well.

For many, this will be far from easy. Sugar-lovers at first may suffer the same kind of torture as chain-smokers trying to give up cigarettes. But dietary fiber does more than diet pills to curb an appetite for sweets, and if you get into the habit of reaching for fruit when you feel sugar-starved, it will help enormously.

The high-fiber way *is the only long-term way to cure sugar addiction.*

Synthetic sweeteners simply substitute one unhealthy practice for another. These sweeteners are pure chemical, without any food value whatsoever, and their long-range cumulative effect may be hazardous to health.

Nor is substituting honey for sugar an answer, since, as noted, honey synthesizes more fat than does white sugar.

After you have achieved your weight-loss goal and want to maintain your new weight, you may again enjoy *light desserts,* those low in sugar or other sweetening—but make sure they contain no more than 1 or 1½ teaspoons of sugar in each serving.

Why are fruits acceptable, since they, too, are fairly high in sugar? Because their natural sugar is not in concentrated form; it is diluted with considerable amounts of moisture and the fruit's fiber will carry off excess sugar. Moreover fruit supplies many important nutritive elements—vitamins, minerals, even some protein—and refined sugar has none of these. This is why I use fruits and fruit juices as a substitute for at least part of the sugar called for in recipes.

In some cases, I use whole-bran cereal as a sugar substitute, since the composition of these cereals is about one-fifth sucrose. Because of the fiber in the bran, most of this sucrose will be carried away and will not remain in the bloodstream.

The Vegetable Answer

Try unusual vegetable combinations such as Spiced Carrots with Mushrooms, or Stir-Fried Eggplant and Green Peppers, pages 37 and 38. Also see Chapter 10.

The following vegetables are outstanding both for low-calorie and high-fiber content:

broccoli   cauliflower
brussels sprouts   celery and celery root
carrots   collard greens

dandelion greens   parsnips
green beans   red cabbage
kale   rutabagas
okra   winter squash

Fruits and Fiber

Some fruits are better fiber sources than others. Black-berries top the list, with other berries not far behind. Apples, pears, apricots, peaches, plums, and fresh pineapple are excellent. Although citrus fruits are not as valuable for fiber as some others, a single large navel orange furnishes twice as much fiber as a bowl of Wheaties.

Protein and the High-Fiber Diet

Obviously doing without sugar will take off pounds, but why cut down on meat? First, because of meat's high fat content. Note from the following charts that even *lean* meats are surprisingly high in fat, while a serving of rib roast of beef may contain as much as 44 grams of fat and two frankfurters 30 grams.

Note in the second chart how much protein is available in some plant foods. Many vegetables contain protein; although it is not a complete or "high quality" protein, when these vegetables are consumed in combination with other protein, they perform much the same function in metabolism. For example, ¾ cup of green peas has 6 grams of protein, 9 medium-sized brussels sprouts, 5 grams, and each of the following 4 grams of protein: 1 ear of corn, ½ cup of collard greens, 1 stalk of broccoli, and 5 or 6 asparagus spears.

Animal Food*	Portion	Grams Protein	Grams Fat	Calories per Serving
hamburger	1 patty	11	15	182
codfish, broiled	3½ ounces	29	5.3	170
tuna, canned	¼ can	14.4	4.2	98
chicken breast	3½ ounces	28.6	6.4	203
lean top round, broiled	3½ ounces	28.6	15.4	261
broiled chuck	3½ ounces	16.2	31.4	352
rib roast	3½ ounces	18.3	44.7	481
loin pork chop	3½ ounces	23.5	35.0	418
baked ham slice	3½ ounces	29.7	10	217
frankfurters	2	14	20-30	248
bologna	3½ ounces	15	16	221
eggs, cooked	2 medium	13	12	162

*All figures are for cooked foods.

Plant Food*	Portion	Grams Protein	Grams Fat	Calories per Serving
millet	¾ cup	9.9	2.9	160
bulgur	¾ cup	8.7	1.4	184
brown rice	⅔ cup	2.5	0.6	135
white rice (converted)	⅔ cup	2.1	0.1	116
macaroni, spaghetti	1 cup	5.0	0.5	192
dried limas	¾ cup	8.2	0.6	207
chickpeas	¾ cup	9.2	2.4	180
soybeans	¾ cup	11.0	5.7	195
white beans	¾ cup	7.8	0.6	177
kidney beans	¾ cup	7.8	0.4	177
lentils	¾ cup	7.8	1.1	159

*All figures are for cooked foods.

Cholesterol, Fat, and Fiber

Medical science has not yet solved the mystery of why blood cholesterol is higher in some individuals than others. Most physicians recommend that patients with a high cholesterol count avoid all animal fats, but a growing number of medical researchers are convinced that *sugar* may be just as responsible as fats for raising cholesterol levels. The body makes its own cholesterol; whether foods rich in cholesterol are more likely to be transformed into cholesterol in the body or whether cholesterol is produced as a result of a complex chemical reaction brought on by other ingredients is not yet known for certain.

In the meantime, the high-fiber diet offers an answer to those who wish to play it safe, because *no plant foods contain cholesterol.* (Nuts, however, are rich in fat, and therefore, anyone concerned with weight control should pass them up.)

Other fats, too, should be avoided with the exception of a limited amount of vegetable oil in the daily diet, important for lubrication and to help in the elimination of wastes. Oil in salad dressings is beneficial to health—as long as the quantity is limited. A lesson to be learned from Chinese cooking is that vegetables *cook more quickly in oil than in water* and, if stirred constantly (the stir-fry technique), do not absorb much oil.

Use less oil or other fat than most recipes call for (in this book, however, I have reduced it to a minimum), and avoid deep-fried foods or those cooked at high heat. The chemical composition of vegetable oils changes at high heat, and they become less digestible.

Heavily refined vegetable oils have no nutritive value except for their fat content. Virgin olive oil is the only one that is not refined at all; Europeans say olive oil is a good source of Vitamin E, and it contains no preservatives. Many health stores now offer corn, safflower, sesame, and soy oils which have been only slightly refined, thereby retaining more natural nutrients, but these and olive oil cost a great deal more than heavily refined oils, a further reason to use them sparingly.

LOW-CALORIE / HIGH-FIBER RECIPES

Strawberries in Orange Juice

1 pint strawberries
2 teaspoons brown sugar
  (optional)

Juice of 1 Florida orange,
  not strained

Wash and trim strawberries, discarding any over-soft or over-ripe berries. Slice in half. Add sugar, let stand while squeezing juice. Remove the seeds and larger pieces of cellulose (skin) from the juice, but not the fruit pulp. Pour over berries. Chill. Makes 4 servings.

Stuffed Appetizer Mushrooms

24 large mushrooms
¼ cup minced onion
1 garlic clove, crushed
3 tablespoons olive oil
½ cup crumbled whole-
  wheat bread
¼ cup chopped sunflower
  kernels

1 tablespoon bran meal
1 tablespoon chopped
  parsley
Salt, pepper
Dash of Tabasco
¼ cup shredded Swiss cheese

Carefully remove stems from mushrooms; chop them if they are not too woody. Sauté onion, garlic, and chopped stems in 2 tablespoons of oil until lightly browned. Add crumbs, stir to blend. Add all the remaining ingredients but the cheese. Stuff mixture into mushroom caps. Brush outside of caps with remaining oil, place in shallow pan, and sprinkle cheese over the stuffing. (This can be done in advance.) Bake in 400° F. oven (preheated) until cheese is melted and mushrooms hot. Serve immediately. Makes 24.

Curried Tuna Pâté

1 envelope unflavored gelatin
¼ cup cold water
1 can (6-7 ounces) tuna, drained
½ green pepper, in ½-inch pieces
¼ cup chopped sunflower kernels
½ lemon, seeded, quartered
1 small onion, quartered
1 teaspoon curry powder
½ teaspoon seasoned salt
½ cup boiling water

Soften gelatin in cold water. Place with all remaining ingredients in blender; beat until well blended but not smooth. Turn mixture into a 2-cup mold; chill until firm. Unmold. Serve as pâté with rye wafers.

Shrimp Apple Dip

1 jar (3½ ounces) tiny Danish or Norwegian shrimp, or 4-ounce can small shrimp, drained
Pinch of powdered ginger
Dash of Tabasco
1 cup (½ 8-ounce package) Neufchâtel cheese
½ apple (not peeled), chopped fine
1 tablespoon freeze-dried chives
3 tablespoons chopped sunflower seeds
¼ cup creamed cottage cheese
1 tablespoon toasted sesame seeds

Mince shrimp; beat to a paste with pestle. Add remaining ingredients, beat until well blended. Keep chilled until ½ hour before serving, then bring to room temperature. Makes about 1 cup.

Okra Vinaigrette

1 pound young okra; or
  10-ounce package frozen
  okra pods
¼ cup vinegar

2 tablespoons oil
2 scallions, thinly sliced
¼ teaspoon salt or seasoned
  salt, or to taste

Cook okra in boiling salted water, *uncovered,* until barely tender, no more than 4 minutes for fresh okra, 2 minutes for frozen. Drain. Add remaining ingredients while warm; chill. Serve as an appetizer or part of a buffet spread. Makes 4 buffet servings, 8 appetizer servings.

Salpichon de Mariscos

2 3½-ounce jars tiny Danish
  or Norwegian shrimp,
  drained
2 small white onions, sliced
  paper-thin, or 6 minced
  scallions
1 medium carrot, quartered,
  cooked 3 minutes, diced

1 cup cooked green peas
¼ cup chopped sweet red
  pepper
¼ cup olive oil
2 tablespoons white or
  sherry vinegar
Salt, other seasonings to taste

Combine all ingredients, marinate for 1 hour before serving. Makes about 8 hors d'oeuvres servings.

Old-Fashioned Vegetable Soup

2 medium onions, chopped
½ cup chopped celery
  or celery root
2 medium carrots, scraped,
  diced fine
2 tablespoons butter
1 can (1 pound) tomatoes
6 cups water
1½ teaspoons salt, or
  2 vegetable bouillon
  cubes

1 parsnip, scraped, diced
1 small potato, peeled,
  diced
1 cup shelled fresh peas or
  cut green beans, or frozen
  peas or beans
½ cup minced parsley
2 sprigs fresh basil, minced

Gently cook chopped onion, celery, and carrots in butter over moderate heat until softened; stir frequently. Do not allow to brown. Transfer to kettle, add remaining ingredients, cook about 20 minutes. Makes 8 servings.

Gazpacho

1 large or 2 small garlic cloves
2 slices oatmeal bread, broken in pieces
½ cup water
¼ cup olive oil
Salt to taste
2 pounds fully ripe tomatoes, peeled, chopped, or 1 large can (1 pound 12 ounces) best quality plum tomatoes
¼ cup minced fresh onion
2 sweet red peppers or pimiento, chopped
2 cups ice-cold water
2 tablespoons sherry or white vinegar
Garnishes: chopped green pepper, minced onion, toasted chopped almonds, croutons (or Wheat Chex)

Crush garlic in bowl, add bread, water, olive oil, and salt; let stand several hours or overnight. Add tomatoes, onion, red sweet pepper or pimiento; beat in blender until pureed. Keep chilled until ready to serve, then add ice-cold water to desired consistency, vinegar, and more salt if needed. At table, pass garnishes in small bowls to be sprinkled over top of soup. (Croutons may be omitted.) Makes 6 servings.

Tuna Cottage Cheese Salad

1 can (6–7 ounces) tuna, drained
½ cup low-fat cottage cheese
1 teaspoon chopped sunflower kernels
1 tablespoon drained capers
1 tablespoon chopped parsley
¼ cup chopped green pepper
¼ cup chopped celery
1 teaspoon Dijon mustard
Salad greens

Combine all ingredients but salad greens, blending well. Serve over shredded greens. Do *not* add dressing. Add a raw apple or pear for dessert, and you have a fine low-calorie lunch.

Makes 4–5 servings. (For 1 or 2 servings, combine equal quantities of tuna and cottage cheese and add the remaining ingredients to taste.)

Beef en Casserole

1½ pounds stewing beef, cut in 1½-inch cubes
2 tablespoons oil
1 medium onion, thickly sliced
3 or 4 white turnips, peeled and cubed
2 parsnips, scraped, cubed
1 large carrot, scraped, cubed
1½ teaspoons salt
2 tablespoons chopped parsley, or ½ teaspoon thyme
2 cups (1 pound) canned tomatoes

Sear beef in oil until browned on all sides; transfer to deep casserole with fitted cover. Add all vegetables but tomatoes to beef, stir to mix. Force tomatoes through sieve, spread over top. Cover casserole; bake in moderate (350° F.) oven for 2–2½ hours. Serve with baked potatoes. Makes 4–6 servings.

Chicken Barbecue

Cut up a broiler-fryer into small pieces, using poultry shears and heavy sharp knife. One hour before cooking, sprinkle chicken on all sides with salt, pepper, powdered cumin, and lemon juice. Place chicken pieces on skewers with zucchini, yellow summer squash, and green pepper squares, cutting the squash into ½-inch slices. Brush generously with sesame oil or olive oil. Broil over charcoal, turning frequently until chicken is well browned. After it has started to brown, brush with the following *Soybean-Parsley Sauce:* coarsely crush in a mortar or blender ¼ cup of toasted soybeans, 1 garlic of clove, ¼ cup of chopped parsley, ¼ cup of sesame or olive oil, and 1 teaspoon of soy sauce. A 3-pound chicken so prepared makes 4–6 servings.

Chinese-Style Chicken Livers

4–6 whole chicken livers
2–3 tablespoons oil
4 scallions, chopped
8–10 fresh mushrooms, sliced
6 white radishes, cut lengthwise, or 2 white turnips, in sticks
8 small spears broccoli, sliced lengthwise

4–5 fresh okra pods, sliced, or ½ package frozen okra
Salt
1 tablespoon soy sauce
1 tablespoon sherry (optional)
2 tablespoons water

Cut chicken livers in half, sauté in oil over high heat until browned on both sides; remove. Lower heat, add scallions and mushrooms; stir-fry until lightly browned. Add remaining vegetables, continue to stir-fry for 3 or 4 minutes. Add more oil if needed. Sprinkle with salt. Add soy sauce, sherry, and water; replace chicken livers, cook about 2 minutes longer. (Vegetables should be half-raw.)

If desired, serve topped with Chinese fried noodles (page 36) or Wheat Chex. Makes 3 or 4 entree servings (for a 1-entree meal).

Carrot-Stuffed Fish

1 4-pound fish (sea bass, sea-trout, large whiting), cleaned
Salt
Lemon juice
1 carrot, scraped, minced
1 apple, unpeeled, chopped
½ cup soft whole-wheat breadcrumbs
1 teaspoon instant minced onion

2 tablespoons minced parsley or fresh dill
1 tablespoon sunflower kernels, chopped
Dijon mustard
1 lemon, sliced
3 tablespoons butter or margarine

Sprinkle fish inside and out with salt and lemon juice; let stand for 10 minutes. Combine carrot, apple, breadcrumbs, onion, parsley, and sunflower kernels; stuff fish with mixture and truss, using small skewers. Place fish in shallow pan; cut slits at 1-inch intervals along back. Rub mustard generously all over. Insert lemon slices in slits, dot with butter. Bake in moderate oven (350° F.) until flesh is quite firm to touch (1–1¼ hours). Allow ½ pound fish per serving.

Poached Fish with Soybean Parsley Sauce

1¾–2 pounds halibut steak
    or turbot, in 1 piece
Salt
Lemon juice

SAUCE:
½ cup toasted soybeans
¼ cup chopped parsley
½ teaspoon garlic powder
1 tablespoon olive oil
½ cup plain yogurt or
    sour cream

Place fish on rack in large roasting pan or deep wide kettle. Sprinkle with salt and lemon juice, let stand 10–30 minutes. Add salted water to pan, cover (use foil if cooked in roasting pan), bring water to a boil, then lower heat and simmer gently 20–25 minutes until fish flakes easily with fork. Serve topped with sauce. Makes 4–6 servings.

To make sauce: Crush soybeans coarsely in mortar, working in parsley and garlic powder, and finally the olive oil and yogurt or sour cream. Makes ½ cup.

Hi-Fiber Shrimp Chow Mein

4 scallions, chopped
1 or 2 garlic cloves, slit
4 tablespoons oil
1 cup celery, sliced at angle
½ cup tender green snap
    beans, cut in pieces
½ cup diced green pepper
½ cup sliced water chestnuts
Salt
1 6-ounce package frozen
    shrimp, thawed

1 tablespoon soy sauce
1 tablespoon whole-wheat or
    soy flour
1 tablespoon sherry
½ cup chicken broth
¼ cup toasted soybeans
Cooked whole-wheat noodles,
    fried, or Wheat Chex

Stir-fry scallions and garlic in 2 tablespoons of oil; when garlic is soft, mash with tines of fork. Add remaining vegetables one at a time in order given; stir-fry each for about 1 minute. Sprinkle with salt. Remove all vegetables to absorbent paper.

Add more oil to pan. Lower heat and stir-fry shrimp just until they turn pink (about 2 minutes). *Do not overcook.* Blend soy sauce, flour, and sherry; thin with chicken broth. Add to shrimp, simmer until sauce is thickened; add soybeans. Replace vegetables and cook about 1 minute. Serve topped with noodles (which can be fried at the same time—see recipe below), or with Wheat Chex. Makes 3 or 4 single-entree servings.

(The above ingredients should serve as a general guideline. Create your own mixture with what you have. By decreasing all ingredients by half, this recipe can be cut to serve 1 or 2 persons.)

Fried Whole-Wheat Noodles

Buy whole-wheat noodles at health store, break in small pieces, cook in boiling salted water until tender; drain. Dry thoroughly. Deep-fry in 1 inch of hot oil until crisp. Drain again on absorbent paper.

Stir-Fried Steak and Vegetables

½ pound top round of beef, cut in thin strips
1 tablespoon cornstarch
1½ tablespoons soy sauce
1 tablespoon sherry
2 or 3 thin slices ginger root, minced
3 tablespoons oil
1 small garlic clove
1 medium onion, cut in sticks
2 large green peppers, cut in squares
1 carrot, very thinly sliced
¾ cup broth

Marinate strips of meat in mixture of cornstarch, soy sauce, sherry, and ginger for 15 minutes or longer. Preheat wok or skillet; when hot, add 1½ tablespoons of oil, garlic, and onion. Stir-fry for 1 or 2 minutes; crush garlic clove. Add remaining vegetables, stir-fry for 2–3 minutes longer; remove from pan.

Clean pan so that no oil remains. Add more oil, heat briefly, then lift meat from marinade and cook ¼ at a time, stirring, for about 3 minutes. Replace vegetables and remaining marinade, cook for 2 minutes longer. Serve immediately. Makes 4 servings.

Salmon Custard

1–pound can salmon
½ cup chopped celery
¼ cup chopped onion
2 tablespoons chopped parsley
¼ cup wheat germ
¼ cup crushed Shredded Wheat
2 tablespoons rye or soy flakes
2 eggs, lightly beaten
1 cup low-fat milk

Empty contents of can of salmon in bowl, bones, skin, and all (the bones provide valuable calcium). Beat in blender until almost pureed. Add remaining ingredients, turn into greased 1-quart casserole; place casserole in shallow pan with water to depth of ½ inch. Bake in moderate oven (350° F.) until knife inserted in center comes out clean (45 minutes–1 hour). Makes 4–6 servings.

Spiced Carrots and Mushrooms

6 large carrots
Salted water
1 cup sliced fresh mushrooms
2–3 tablespoons butter or margarine
Salt
½ teaspoon Chinese 5-spice powder*
½ cup chopped parsley

Scrape carrots, cut each in half, then in quarters. Cook in salted water until barely tender (4–5 minutes). Drain. Meantime sauté mushrooms in butter until lightly browned; sprinkle

*If Chinese 5-spice mixture is not available, use pumpkin pie spice (cinnamon, nutmeg, cloves, ginger) and crushed fennel or anise, a good pinch of each.

with salt. Add the 5-spice powder, parsley, and cooked carrots; continue to cook covered over low heat until carrots are heated through. Keep warm until time to serve. Makes 4–6 servings.

Stir-Fried Eggplant and Green Pepper

2 Italian eggplant, or
 ½ larger eggplant
1 green pepper
3 tablespoons oil

2 white radishes, or 1 white turnip, cut in sticks
Salt

The tiny eggplant called Italian are best for this dish: simply slice thin, then cut slices in half or quarters (do not peel). For a larger eggplant, cut in thin crosswise slices, then cut into ½-inch pieces. The green pepper should be cut in 1-inch squares. Heat oil, add the eggplant, green pepper, and radish or turnip, sprinkle with salt, and stir-fry until tender. Move continuously with spatula to keep from sticking and to prevent eggplant from absorbing too much oil. Cook for about 4–5 minutes. An excellent dish for a meatless meal, it makes 2 or 3 entree servings, 4–6 side servings.

Sweet and Sour Cabbage

4 cups shredded cabbage
1 large carrot, scraped,
 grated
1 large or 2 small onions,
 thinly sliced
Grated rind and juice of
 ½ lemon

4 apples, cored, diced
¼ cup apple juice
1 teaspoon caraway seeds
½ cup currants or raisins
Pinch of allspice or cloves

Place all ingredients in large saucepan or skillet, cover, and bring to a boil over low heat; cook just until cabbage is tender (about 8 minutes). Serve with a little of juice spooned over it. Excellent with baked potato and baked acorn squash as a wintertime supper. Makes 6 servings.

Eggs Divan

1 bunch fresh broccoli
6 hard-cooked eggs
1 3-ounce can sliced mushrooms
1 10½-ounce can cream of chicken soup (condensed)
1 cup low-fat milk
1 tablespoon bran meal

1 3- or 4-ounce can sliced mushrooms, drained
½ cup shredded Swiss cheese
1½ cups Wheat Chex crushed to ¾ cup
2 tablespoons butter
½ teaspoon seasoned salt

Trim broccoli and cut into 12–16 spears of approximately the same size, slicing some stems in center if necessary. (Save leaves and lower stems to cook as a separate vegetable.) Cook in boiling salted water, uncovered, for about 4 minutes; drain. Arrange over bottom of buttered shallow casserole.

Chop hard-cooked eggs. Combine soup, milk, bran, and liquid from canned mushrooms. Place eggs, mushroom slices, and sauce over the broccoli; add ¼ cup of cheese.

Stir-fry crushed cereal in butter; add seasoned salt and remaining cheese. Spread over sauce. (This can be prepared in advance.) Bake in moderate (350° F.) oven until top is browned and sauce bubbling (about ½ hour). Makes 6 servings.

Chicken Divan

Use 1 cup of cooked sliced chicken instead of eggs.

Celery Cabbage and Green Pepper

Cut celery cabbage into 2-inch lengths; combine with a more or less equal quantity of green pepper cut into squares and some chopped scallion. Stir-fry in a little oil until softened but still crisp (about 3 minutes). Season with soy sauce instead of salt. Serve as a side dish.

Quick Frozen Vegetable Medley

1 10-ounce package frozen broccoli spears
1 10-ounce package frozen cauliflower
2 tablespoons oil
1 10-ounce package frozen baby limas
½ cup chopped onion
1 can (8 ounces) stewed tomatoes
1 chicken or vegetable bouillon cube
Salt to taste

Let frozen vegetables stand at room temperature until partially thawed, *or* place in bowls, cover with boiling water, let stand a few minutes, then drain. Heat oil in skillet; add limas first, stir-fry for 1 minute, add onion, stir-fry until lightly browned, then add broccoli, cauliflower (in that order), stirring to mix with onion. Add tomato, bouillon cube, and a little salt. Simmer for 5 minutes. Taste; adjust seasoning. **Makes 8 servings.**

Vegetarian Chef's Salad

1 cup shredded carrots
1 cup cooked green beans
1 cup chopped cooked beets
Shredded romaine
Watercress sprigs
¼ cup toasted soybeans
1 teaspoon fennel seeds
4 hard-cooked eggs, cut in wedges
½ cup black olives (pitted)
12 cherry tomatoes
Oil-Vinegar Dressing

Arrange vegetables in separate bowls; moisten each with dressing, just enough to "wet" the vegetables. Arrange romaine (and any other desired salad greens) in salad bowl; place piles of marinated vegetables over the salad greens. Decorate with watercress, sprinkle with soybeans and fennel seeds. Arrange egg wedges, olives, and tomato around the top. Toss to serve, adding a little more dressing if needed. **Makes 6 entree salad servings.**

Chinese Carrot Salad

4 small carrots, scraped,
   shredded
1 cup thin-sliced chopped
   celery cabbage
2 thin slices ginger root,
   minced

4 water chestnuts, sliced
Fresh bean sprouts
Salt, MSG to taste
2 tablespoons soy sauce
1 tablespoon vinegar

Combine all ingredients; marinate 1 hour before serving.
Makes 4–6 servings.

Pachadi
(East Indian Salad)

1 cup shredded green
   cabbage
1 cup grated carrots
1 cup thin-sliced cucumber
   (not peeled)
2 green chili peppers, cut in
   slivers
1 cup thinly sliced onion
   or chopped scallions

Salt to taste
1 cup plain yogurt
½ teaspoon paprika
1 tablespoon chopped fresh
   coriander or ground
   coriander seeds
Watercress sprigs

Combine all ingredients but watercress; let stand until time to
serve, then garnish with watercress. Makes 6 servings.

Raspberry Yogurt Parfait

1 10-ounce package frozen
   red raspberries
½ cup plain yogurt
1 peach, peeled, sliced

1 navel orange, chopped
½ cup blueberries or
   strawberries

Defrost raspberries; drain, saving juice. Blend a little of the
juice with the yogurt. Combine the four kinds of fruit; place
in sherbet dishes and top with the raspberry-sweetened yogurt.
Makes 4 or 5 servings.

Other low-calorie/high-fiber recipes will be found throughout this book, marked with this sign: LC. Note especially the salads and fruit desserts.

Suggested low-calorie menus will also be found on pages 236–240.

CHAPTER 4

Bread and Cereals: The Heart of the Matter

For untold centuries bread was considered "the staff of life" because the crudely ground cereals of which it was made contained so many important nutrients—including protein. When the rolling mills technique of refining wheat flour was perfected a century ago, not everyone hailed the invention. As already mentioned, Seventh Day Adventists launched a "health food" campaign, introducing whole-grain breakfast cereals to replace the lost bran removed in the milling process. Ironically, today at least half of the ready-to-eat breakfast cereals in supermarket distribution are quite as harmful as the overrefined white flour they were created to combat—because of their high sugar content and use of refined rather than whole-grain cereals.

A study by Dr. Ira Shannon, director of the Oral Disease Research Laboratory at the Houston Veterans Administration, points up this dietary threat. In an article that appeared in the September–October issue of the *Journal of Dentistry for Children,** Dr. Shannon listed the leading breakfast cereals and the amount of sucrose his researchers had found each contained. Here are some from an extensive list:

	% sucrose (sugar)
Shredded Wheat (large biscuit)	1.0
Shredded Wheat (spoon size)	1.3
Cheerios	2.2
Wheat Chex	2.6
Wheaties	4.7
Raisin Bran (Kellogg)	10.6
Heartland (with raisins)	13.5
Granola (with dates or raisins)	14.5

*As quoted by Marian Burros in the Washington *Post,* April 3, 1975.

43

40% Bran Flakes (Post)	15.8
40% Bran Flakes (Kellogg)	16.2
100% Bran (Nabisco)	18.4
All Bran (Kellogg)	20.0
Bran Buds	20.2
Fortified Oat Flakes	22.2
Frosted Mini Wheats	33.6
Cocoa Puffs	43.0
Frosted Flakes	44.2
Pink Panther	49.2
Super Orange Crisp	68.0

Of all the cereals analyzed, Dr. Shannon found that twenty-eight brands in national distribution contained 40 percent or more sucrose—the average amount of sucrose in candies is only 37.1 percent. (A certain amount of sucrose occurs naturally in cereal grains, which explains why Shredded Wheat with no sugar added could contain 1 percent.)

Cereals for Breakfast

The idea of starting the day with a bowl of whole-grain cereals is as valid as ever—provided the cereals chosen are low in sucrose. Cereal *plus* milk can supply one-fourth of the day's protein requirements, and when dried or fresh fruits are added, it is possible to have as much as a third of the day's fiber requirements in one bowl. (Incidentally, dried currants are ideal for sprinkling over breakfast cereal: they are almost twice as high in fiber as raisins, yet are lower in calories.)

Instead of buying granola mixtures, why not create your own? You can cut down on calories and save money, too.

Easy Granola

Create your own granola mixture from one or more low-sucrose ready-to-eat breakfast cereals, adding seeds or whole grains and currants or other dried fruits. Here are some examples to get you started:

1. Combine crumbled Shredded Wheat, Wheat Chex, a few

flakes of rolled rye, 1 teaspoon (or less) of buckwheat grains, and 1 or 2 teaspoons of dried currants.

2. Combine Wheaties, Cheerios, and either 40% Bran Flakes or one of the whole-bran cereals, plus 1 teaspoon of triticale flakes, shredded coconut (unsweetened), sunflower kernels, and raisins.

3. Combine a Shredded Wheat biscuit with chopped prunes or dates, some Kretchmer wheat germ *or* Grape-Nuts, and pure bran meal.

4. Toast oatmeal in oven or stir-fry it in a teaspoonful of oil until lightly browned; add All Bran or 100% Bran, currants or raisins, rolled wheat flakes (whole-grain) and buckwheat grains. Serve topped with sliced bananas and milk.

Quick Fruit Granola

¼ cup chopped dates
½ cup dried currants
½ cup unsweetened dried coconut
¼ cup sunflower kernels
¼ cup rye flakes

1 cup 40% Bran Flakes
1 cup spoon-size Shredded Wheat
1 cup Cheerios
1 cup Wheat Chex
¼ cup toasted soybeans

Dates can be purchased already chopped but these "nuggets" have been sugared and therefore are less desirable than regular pitted dates that you chop yourself. Combine all ingredients, mix well, then divide into serving-size portions, and "bag" separately, tying each with metal twists. Makes 7 portions.

Fruited Porridge

Make porridge with oatmeal, Wheatena, Ralston, stone-ground cornmeal, Roman Meal (available on the West Coast), or millet meal. As the porridge cooks, stir in a handful of any of the following:

dried currants
chopped dates
raisins
chopped apples
chopped dried apricots

chopped prunes
plus
wheat germ
whole-bran cereal
shredded coconut *or* chopped peanuts

Hi-Fiber Cornmeal Mush

4 cups water
1 teaspoon salt
1 cup stone-ground cornmeal
¼ cup bran meal

¼ cup wheat germ
Soy or whole-wheat flour
2 tablespoons shortening

Grease a small loaf pan. Place water and salt in large saucepan, bring to a rapid boil, then slowly stir in mixture of cornmeal, bran, and wheat germ, stirring constantly about 5 minutes. Lower heat, cover, cook about 20 minutes longer, or until thick and free from lumps. (You may find it easier to complete cooking in top of double boiler.) Pour into loaf pan, chill overnight. For breakfast, unmold, cut in ¼-inch slices, dust on both sides with flour, then fry in hot fat until well browned on both sides. Makes 10–12 servings. (Keeps well in refrigerator if it is not all used at once.)

Cereals for Quick Breads

The word "cereal" applies to all edible grains with nutritive value, whether eaten raw, cooked as porridge, or ground into flour or meal. But not all flours from cereals are suitable for baking. Wheat flour, because of its gluten content, produces the best baked products—especially white flour. The gluten in the bran-free white flour expands like a balloon, as gases form from yeast action. This is why bakers and pastry cooks prefer using white flour, and why most "whole-wheat" breads are made with half white flour. Whether yeast-raised or "quick breads," those made with whole-grain flour tend to be heavier in texture and more compact. But once you develop a taste for hearty whole-grain breads, white bread seems utterly blah.

The following terms, applied to various forms of white flour, unless otherwise noted, need to be understood before purchasing flour for baking.

All-purpose flour, always a white flour made from wheat, is a mixture of hard and soft varieties of wheat. (All unbleached flour is "all-purpose.") It is suitable for breads, pie crust, pastas, and numerous other uses.

Cake flour is white flour milled from soft varieties of wheat, low in gluten. It has been very highly refined.

Whole-wheat pastry flour is also made from soft wheat and *its fiber content is identical to that of white all-purpose flour.*

"Enriched" flours have had vitamin and mineral components added to make up in part for all the nutrients taken away.

Bleached flour has been processed to give the flour snowy whiteness, but the bleaching destroys vitamins.

Unbleached flour is always white, but not quite so refined, and it retains more vitamins and other nutritive elements.

Instantized or instant-type flours have been even more refined than "all-purpose" in order to dissolve instantly in liquids and not require sifting. But they've lost still more food value in the process.

Self-rising flours have had a leavening agent (soda, baking powder, or another chemical) and salt added. There are self-rising cake flours, self-rising bread flours, and also self-rising cornmeal (both stone-ground and degermed). Use self-rising flours *only* for making quick breads and cakes, never in recipes that require yeast or any which do not need a leavener.

Rye flour is the only other cereal grain besides wheat that may be used *by itself* for making yeast breads. Dark rye flour is traditionally used in northern Europe and Russia for peasant "black breads." There are three types of rye flour: light, medium, and dark, the latter sometimes labeled "100 percent rye." Rye flour and cornmeal are frequently used together in breads, but cornmeal by itself is suitable only for quick breads or pancakes, not for yeast-raised breads.

Buckwheat flour, too, is used chiefly in combination with other flours. It is increasingly hard to find. Products made with it tend to have an unattractive gray color unless darkened with molasses.

Soy flour, also used in combination with other flours, is valued for its high protein and fiber content and is an outstanding source of calcium and phosphorus. It does not contain enough gluten for very satisfactory baked goods.

Carob "flour" is not a flour but a powder, ground from the pod of the carob tree. It is used like cocoa, which it resembles in color and flavor, though it has more natural sweetness.

Other "flours" in the following list also are to be used only in combinations for baking, although all are sufficiently high in starch to be used as "binders" for sauces and croquettes.

Oatmeal, or *rolled oats,* is a good source of protein and a moderate source of fiber. It, too, must be used in combination with flours containing gluten. *Potato* and *rice* flour are used only as thickeners, not for baking.

(The *USDA Handbook* mentions an oat flakes product processed from toasted wheat germ and soy grits with a 20 percent protein content and 3.5 percent fiber content, but I have been unable to locate it.)

Fiber Percentages of Flours

whole-wheat all-purpose flour	2.3
whole-wheat pastry flour	0.4
white all-purpose flour (bleached or unbleached)	0.4
gluten flour	0.4
pure bran meal (wheat)	9.1–12
soy flour	2.3–2.5
rye flour, dark	2.4
medium	1.2
light	0.4
cornmeal, whole ground	1.6
bolted	1.0
degermed (regular commercial), yellow and white	0.7
sunflower seed flour	4.6
rolled oats or oatmeal	1.2
instant or quick-cooking	0.7
buckwheat flour	1.6
buckwheat pancake mix	1.4
lima bean flour	2.0
carob powder	7.7

Biscuits and Muffins

Supplement flours low in fiber content with bran meal or whole-bran cereal (keeping in mind the latter's sugar content —use only when added sweetness is desired).

In any bran muffin recipe, you can use ¼ cup of molasses in place of ½ cup of sugar, and add dried fruit for sweetening.

If you use commercial biscuit mix, refrigerator biscuits, or any similar mix made with refined flour, add bran meal or whole-bran cereal. (Knead bran into refrigerator biscuits, then reshape.)

The most useful recipe in this section is for Refrigerator Bran Muffins. The batter keeps in the refrigerator for days, even weeks, and you spoon out only as much as you want at a time.

Recipes with a 12-muffin yield may be baked ahead, bagged in 3- or 4-muffin portions, frozen, then reheated when needed.

Jane Mengenhauser's Refrigerator Bran Muffins

¼ cup molasses

½ cup oil or vegetable shortening

2 eggs

2½ cups unbleached all-
purpose flour

2½ teaspoons soda

½ teaspoon salt

2 cups buttermilk

1 cup unsweetened apple
juice, heated almost to
boiling

1 cup Nabisco 100% Bran

¾ cup chopped prunes, currants, or mixed dried fruit

2 cups Kellogg's All Bran

Combine molasses and oil or shortening; beat in eggs one at a time. Add flour, soda, salt, and buttermilk; mix until smooth. Pour *hot* apple juice over the 100% Bran; let stand until cereal has absorbed the liquid and cooled slightly. Blend into batter. Add fruit and the All Bran. Mix well.

Refrigerate batter, covered, to be used as needed. When ready to use, simply dip batter into greased muffin tins *without stirring.* Fill muffin cups almost full. Bake in an oven preheated to 400° F. (hot) for about 20 minutes. Batter will keep up to six weeks in the refrigerator.

Pineapple Bran Muffins

1 cup unbleached all-purpose
flour

½ teaspoon salt

2 teaspoons baking powder

1 cup whole-bran breakfast
cereal

1 cup milk

2 tablespoons oil

½ cup well-drained crushed
unsweetened pineapple

1 egg, beaten

Prepare two 6-cup muffin tins (if Teflon-coated they need not be greased). Combine flour, salt, and baking powder; stir in the bran, then milk and oil, then the pineapple and egg. Beat just until dry ingredients are thoroughly moistened; spoon into muffin cups. Bake in preheated 400° F. (hot) oven for 20–25 minutes, or until golden and pulling away from sides of cups. Makes 12. (Half can be frozen for another breakfast.)

Orange Date Muffins

½ cup unbleached flour
1½ cups whole-wheat flour
3 teaspoons baking powder
½ teaspoon salt
1 tablespoon brown sugar

2 teaspoons grated orange rind
1 egg, beaten
3 tablespoons oil
¾ cup orange juice
½ cup chopped dates

Combine dry ingredients and orange rind. Beat together egg, oil, and orange juice. Stir mixture quickly into dry ingredients; add dates. Spoon into 12 prepared muffin cups, filling ⅔ full. Bake in oven preheated to 425° F. for 20–25 minutes. Remove from tins immediately; serve hot. Makes 12.

Carrot Muffins

2 cups whole-wheat flour
½ teaspoon salt
2 teaspoons baking powder
1 tablespoon brown sugar
1 tablespoon grated lemon rind

1 egg
¼ cup oil
½ cup milk
½ cup shredded raw carrots
¼ cup chopped peanuts or currants (optional)

Combine everything in mixing bowl at once; stir just to moisten flour completely. Spoon into 12 greased (or Teflon-coated) muffin cups. Bake in oven preheated to 400° F. for 20 minutes, or until nicely browned and pulling away from sides. Serve hot. Makes 12.

Blueberry Corn Muffins

1½ cups stone-ground cornmeal
½ cup unbleached all-
 purpose flour
3 teaspoons baking powder
1 teaspoon salt
1 tablespoon bran meal

2 tablespoons clover or
 wildflower honey
1 egg
1 cup low-fat milk
2 tablespoons oil or melted
 butter or margarine
1 cup fresh blueberries

Combine cornmeal, flour, baking powder, salt, and bran in mixing bowl. Beat together honey, egg, milk, and oil or butter; add to the cornmeal mixture and stir until flour is completely moistened. Stir in berries. Spoon into greased (or Teflon-coated) muffin cups. Bake in oven preheated to 400° F. for 20–25 minutes, or until nicely browned and pulling from sides. Makes 12.

Date Corn Muffins

Prepare as for Blueberry Corn Muffins but add only 1 table-spoon of honey and substitute 1 cup of chopped pitted dates for the blueberries.

PANCAKES AND WAFFLES

Many pancake mixes, including some made with soy flour, can be found in health stores. You can also make your own ready "mix" by combining flour, baking powder (or soda), and salt; when you want to make pancakes, just add egg, oil, and liquid.

Any of the following may be added to pancake batter: chopped nuts, chopped unpeeled apple, chopped cooked ham or bacon, fresh blueberries, vegetable protein "bacon bits," buckwheat grains, and sunflower kernels.

For toppings, instead of "maple-flavored syrup" (which is nothing more than concentrated sucrose artificially flavored), use blackberry or raspberry jam, fruit nut conserve, a blend of yogurt and honey, or honey and orange juice heated to-

gether until syrupy. Or top cakes or waffles with one of the
following:

Honey Coconut Topping

Combine ½ cup of honey with ½ cup of unsweetened shredded
coconut and 1 tablespoon of butter or margarine. Heat just
until well blended; serve hot. Makes 1 cup.

Orange Nut Syrup

Combine ¼ cup each of frozen orange juice concentrate,
molasses, and light brown sugar; add 2 tablespoons of butter, a
little grated orange rind, and 2 tablespoons of chopped toasted
almonds. Heat until thick and well blended. Serve warm.
Makes a little less than 1 cup.

Honey Butter

Blend 3 tablespoons of honey into ½ pound of softened butter.
Keep in small covered crock in refrigerator to use as wanted.
For added fiber, when using the honey butter on pancakes or
waffles, pass a bowl of chopped nuts or wheat germ to sprinkle
over the melting butter.

Buckwheat Pancakes and Sausages

¾ cup buckwheat flour	2 eggs
½ cup whole-wheat flour	1–2 tablespoons light
1 tablespoon buckwheat	molasses
grains	1 tablespoon oil or shortening
1 teaspoon soda	¾–1 cup buttermilk
½ teaspoon salt	

Sausage links (pork or vegetable protein)

Combine the flours and buckwheat grains, soda, and salt. Beat
eggs in mixing bowl, add molasses, oil, and ¾ cup of buttermilk. Stir in flour mixture until all flour is moistened (do not
beat). If too stiff, add a little more liquid, but the batter
should be fairly thick. Let batter stand about 10 minutes before making cakes.

Meantime, fry the sausages. Pure pork sausages are traditional, but for vegetarians or those on low-cholesterol diets, Morningstar or other vegetable protein sausages may be served instead. When browned on all sides, remove the sausages, add ¾ cup of water to the pan drippings, simmer, stirring up any browned bits from the pan, and reduce to ½ cup. Use this over the pancakes instead of syrup.

Bake cakes on a lightly greased griddle in the usual way. Makes about 10 thick pancakes.

Buckwheat Pecan Pancakes or Waffles

Prepare batter as above but instead of buckwheat grains, add ½ cup of chopped pecans. Separate the eggs, putting aside the whites. Increase liquid to 1 (or 1¼) cup, and increase shortening to 3 tablespoons.

100 Percent Whole-Wheat Pancakes

1 teaspoon baking soda	1 tablespoon molasses
1 cup whole-wheat flour	1 cup buttermilk
½ teaspoon salt	1 tablespoon oil
1 egg	

Combine soda, flour, and salt in mixing bowl; make a well in the center. Break egg in bowl, beat until smooth; then add molasses, buttermilk, and oil, and gradually stir flour into liquid ingredients until flour is completely moistened. Do not overbeat. Let stand for 5–10 minutes while heating griddle. Turn pancakes as soon as they are puffed and full of bubbles. Serve topped with butter and gooseberry or red raspberry jam. Makes about 12 pancakes.

Fruit Nut Pancakes

To recipe for 100 percent Whole-Wheat Pancakes, add ½ cup of chopped pitted prunes or other dried fruit, ¼ cup of chopped walnuts, and 2 tablespoons of rolled rye flakes. Increase liquid to 1½ cups of buttermilk. Serve for lunch topped with cottage cheese.

Bran Pancakes

1 cup All Bran cereal
¼ cup hot water
1 cup buttermilk pancake mix

1 egg, beaten
1 cup water or low-fat milk
1 tablespoon oil

Place cereal in small bowl, add hot water, and let stand until water is absorbed. In another bowl, combine pancake mix, egg, water or milk, and oil; beat just to moisten flour. Stir in softened cereal. Bake pancakes on the griddle in usual way. Makes about 20 pancakes.

Spider Corn Cakes

1½ cups stone-ground yellow cornmeal
1 teaspoon baking soda
1 teaspoon salt

2 eggs, beaten
2 cups buttermilk
2 tablespoons butter or margarine, melted

Mix cornmeal with soda and salt; add eggs, buttermilk, and 1 tablespoon of melted butter. Stir just to blend well, but do not beat. Let stand for 5 minutes while heating griddle. Brush griddle with part of remaining butter or margarine; drop batter on griddle in the usual way, but allow more cooking time. Turn when cakes have puffed up and are lightly browned on bottom. Serve topped with light molasses. Makes about 12 pancakes.

Carob Waffles

These look and taste like chocolate waffles and may be served for dessert topped with sour cream, or for brunch (following unsweetened fruit cup) accompanied by crisp bacon.

½ cup carob powder
1 cup soya-carob special blend flour, or all-purpose flour
½ teaspoon salt
1 tablespoon bran meal (optional)

2 tablespoons brown sugar
1½ teaspoons baking powder
2 eggs, separated
2 tablespoons oil
1¾ cups milk
¼ cup chopped walnuts (optional)

Combine first 6 ingredients, blend well. Beat egg whites until stiff, set aside. To flour mixture, add oil, egg yolks, and milk and beat just until well blended. Stir in nuts, then the beaten egg whites. Bake in preheated waffle iron (lightly greased for first batch of waffles). Serve topped with sour cream. Makes about 16 quarters or 4 servings.

Carob Pancakes

Use the same ingredients but do not separate eggs and use only 1 tablespoon of oil. Bake on griddle like any pancakes. Serve topped with sour cream or yogurt.

Whole-Wheat French Toast

Dip slices of whole-wheat bread into a mixture of 1 beaten egg, ¼ cup of milk, and ¼ teaspoon of salt. This is enough for 2–3 slices of bread; double for 4–6 slices. Fry in hot melted butter or margarine, turning to brown on each side. Serve topped with a mixture of yogurt and honey and a sprinkling of whole-bran cereal (optional), or with pure maple syrup and toasted almonds.

QUICK LOAF BREADS

For the first of the following recipes, use a 9x5x3-inch loaf pan; grease well. These quick loaves are rather sweet, suitable for serving with tea. The first is a truly scrumptious recipe, also good for sandwiches, with a cottage cheese or cream cheese filling.

Quick Bran Loaf

2 cups unsifted whole-wheat flour
2 cups 100% Bran Flakes
1½ teaspoons baking powder
1 teaspoon baking soda
1 teaspoon salt
¼ cup crushed nuts

2 eggs
2 tablespoons light molasses
3 tablespoons margarine
2 cups unsweetened apple juice
1 teaspoon grated orange rind

Preheat oven to 375° F. Grease 9x5x3-inch loaf pan. Combine in mixing bowl the flour, cereal, baking powder, soda, salt, and nuts. Make a well in the center, break in eggs, and beat to blend. Add molasses, margarine (does not need to be melted), apple juice, and grated orange rind. Beat just until flour is completely moistened. Spoon batter into loaf pan. Let stand on top of stove for 5 minutes, then bake about 1 hour, or until tester inserted in center comes out clean. Makes 1 large loaf. May be served warm or cold.

Cranberry Nut Bread

1 cup unbleached all-purpose flour
2 teaspoons baking powder
1 teaspoon salt
¼ teaspoon baking soda
¾ cup whole-wheat flour
¼ cup soy flour
3 tablespoons brown sugar
1 egg, beaten

3 tablespoons oil
1 teaspoon grated orange rind
¾ cup orange juice
¾ cup fresh cranberries, put through grinder
½ cup chopped walnuts
½ cup chopped pitted prunes

Grease bottom of loaf pan. Sift together white flour, baking powder, salt, and soda, place in mixing bowl. Stir in whole-wheat and soy flour and sugar. Make a well in the center, add egg, oil, grated rind and juice. Stir just to moisten flour thoroughly. Drain cranberries thoroughly, mix with nuts and prunes, and stir into batter. Turn batter into loaf pan, bake in oven preheated to 350° F. for 1 hour, or until bread starts to pull away from sides and cake tester inserted in center comes out clean. Cool in pan for 10 minutes, then turn out on rack. When cold, wrap in foil or plastic and chill overnight. Slice while chilled, but for best flavor, return to room temperature before serving. Makes 1 loaf.

Possible variations: Instead of walnuts, add ½ cup of crushed Wheat Chex (crushed before measuring) and ¼ cup of chopped sunflower kernels. Or omit prunes, add ¼ cup of flaked coconut, ¼ cup of whole-bran cereal, and ¼ cup of chopped dates.

Banana Orange Bread

½ cup whole-bran cereal
1 cup orange juice
1 cup mashed banana
2 tablespoons light molasses
1 cup unbleached all-purpose flour
1 teaspoon grated orange rind
1 tablespoon baking powder

¼ cup instant dried milk (optional)
½ teaspoon salt
2 eggs
¼ cup margarine or oil
¼ cup shredded coconut
½ cup toasted almonds or sunflower kernels

Place cereal in bowl, add orange juice, and let stand until softened. Mix mashed banana and molasses. Combine in mixing bowl the flour, grated rind, baking powder, dried milk, and salt. Separately beat together eggs, margarine or oil, and banana mixture; add this to flour mixture with softened cereal, coconut, and nuts; stir just until dry ingredients are thoroughly moistened. Pour into greased 8x4x2½-inch (approximately) loaf pan. Bake in moderate oven (350° F.) for 50–55 minutes, or until tester inserted in center comes out clean. Cool in pan for 10 minutes, then turn out on rack. When cold, wrap in foil or plastic, chill overnight before slicing, then return to room temperature before serving. Makes 1 loaf.

MISCELLANEOUS QUICK BREADS

Wheat Tortillas

2 cups whole-wheat flour
1 teaspoon salt
½ teaspoon baking soda

⅓ cup oil
1 cup water

Combine flour, salt, and soda; stir in oil and water and mix well. With fingers and palms of hands, knead mixture until smooth, then form 12 balls of equal size. Press each ball between 2 sheets of waxed paper to make circles about 5 inches in diameter. Bake on hot *ungreased* griddle until lightly browned on each side. Makes 12.

Indian Chapati

1½ cups whole-wheat flour	1 tablespoon oil
1 teaspoon salt	⅓ cup cold water

Mix flour, salt, and oil thoroughly; add water a little at a time to make a soft dough. Divide into 8 pieces, roll out each as thin as possible between sheets of waxed paper, to approximately 8 inches in diameter. Remove upper sheet of paper; cover all chapati with a damp towel for 20 minutes. Bake one at a time on an *ungreased* griddle, turning frequently until crisp and lightly browned. Push down around the edges with a spatula as they cook so that they puff in center. Cool before serving; they will become quite crisp. Serve with curried dishes instead of bread. Makes 8.

Boston Brown Bread

This, the traditional New England recipe, is neither a quick bread nor a raised yeast bread, but steamed. However, the same recipe can be baked in the oven (see the following instructions). It will slice easier when cold, but always reheat it, wrapped in foil, before serving.

1 cup rye flour	¼ cup dark molasses
1 cup stone-ground cornmeal	2 cups buttermilk
1 cup whole-wheat flour	2 metal cans for molds, or 1-
2 teaspoons baking soda	quart steam mold
1 teaspoon salt	

First prepare the molds. Two empty tin cans (1 pound size) with top carefully removed (no jagged edges) may be used. Grease inside thoroughly. In mixing bowl, combine all dry ingredients, stir in molasses and buttermilk until fairly smooth (do not beat). Pour mixture into mold or molds; do not fill more than ⅔ full. Cover top of each with buttered brown or waxed paper (buttered side toward the batter) and tie outside with string or secure with rubber band. (If steam mold has its own cover, merely grease inside of cover.) Place on trivet or rack inside a large kettle with water halfway up the sides of the molds. Cover and steam for 3½ hours. Do not remove molds from kettle until water has cooled, and do not remove bread from molds until cold. Run a knife around sides, then turn out. Reheat wrapped in foil or inside a towel or napkin in warming oven before serving. Makes 2 small or 1 large loaf.

To bake Boston Brown Bread: Prepare exactly as in recipe above, filling molds ⅔ full, *or* spread batter in greased 9x5x3-inch loaf pan. Place molds or pan in a larger pan with *hot* water halfway up sides. Cover molds or pan tightly. Bake 35–45 minutes, or until tester inserted in center comes out clean. (It's better to give the bread more rather than less time—because it is steamed, longer baking will not dry it out.) Cool completely before removing from cans or pan.

Fruited Boston Brown Bread

Add ½ cup of chopped dates or ½ cup of currants to above batter. This batter will fill 3 1-pound cans or a 6-cup mold.

Baking with Yeast

In the last few years, many new bread-making techniques have been introduced. In the Standard Brands test kitchens, the rapid-mix, no-dissolve method of first blending active dry yeast with flour and other dry ingredients is considered a "breakthrough." Instead of the traditional way of dissolving yeast first in lukewarm water, hot water is added to the mix. Another new technique recently has been introduced by Mrs. Gloria Falkenburg in her "Breadmake" classes in the Washington, D.C., area; this cuts preparation time somewhat by eliminating the second rising of the dough. But no one should attempt to make yeast-raised breads in a hurry—it simply can't be done.

Whole-grain flours give less volume than white flour, so, when using them, it is usually best to use smaller loaf pans, the 8x4x2-inch size (approximate measure). Kneading is very important; if not kneaded sufficiently, bread has poor volume and a coarse texture. Whole-grain breads are always coarser and more crumbly than white, but have far more flavor.

Sifting flour before measuring is not necessary, no matter what kind of flour is used. The purpose of sifting flour is to ensure accurate measurements, but in bread-making there are so many variables—such as the density of the flour and the humidity and temperature, that the exact amount of flour needed may vary considerably from one time to another. Knowing how much flour is enough is a question of "feel." You add flour until the dough "comes away from the bowl," leaving the sides almost clean. Do not add more flour as you knead; just flour your hands and the countertop or board.

One recipe for bread made entirely with whole-wheat flour follows, but expect more satisfactory results (at first, anyway) when using a combination of flours.

An *unlighted* oven is a good spot in which to place dough for rising. In a gas oven the pilot light may provide enough warmth, but if you have an electric stove, you should turn on the oven for a minute, then turn off the heat. Another good place is in a corner next to the stove; the bowl containing the dough should be covered with a terrycloth towel to keep in the warmth. But remember that if the dough rises too fast or becomes too high, it may fall during baking.

Before starting, get out all the necessary equipment: mixing bowl, wooden spoon, measuring cups and spoons, loaf pans, and a rack for cooling breads.

Oil or other fat added to dough helps keep bread fresh longer but is not essential. Normally, neither oil nor sugar is added to French-type breads. For a very crisp crust, brush shaped dough with a mixture of egg white and water (1 unbeaten egg white, 1 tablespoon of water); brush half the mixture over dough before baking, the rest halfway through. For a glossy crust, brush with margarine while the bread is still warm.

The more yeast used in proportion to flour, the faster the dough rises, but for some breads, longer, slower rising is preferred for a crisper exterior.

Golden Grain Bread

This is one of the high-fiber bread recipes demonstrated at Gloria Falkenburg's popular "Breadmake" classes.

1½ cups unbleached flour
½ cup rolled oats
1 teaspoon salt
1 package active dry yeast (or 1 scant tablespoon)
1 tablespoon oil

2 tablespoons light molasses
1⅔ cups hot water (120–130°)
1¾–2 cups whole-wheat flour
2 8½x4x2½-inch pans

Place in mixing bowl the unbleached flour, oats, salt, and undissolved yeast; mix well. Add oil, then molasses, and stir to blend. Turn on hot-water tap and let it run until water is quite hot but not scalding. Add water to flour-yeast mixture and beat vigorously by hand or with electric mixer for 2 minutes. Stir in 1½ cups of whole-wheat flour. Let batter rest for 3–4 minutes. Add ¼–½ cup more whole-wheat flour until dough comes away from sides of bowl and will stick to spoon in one piece that can be lifted up.

Lightly dust countertop or breadboard with flour and dust flour over hands. Begin to knead: pick up dough, fold over, and with the heel of the hand press down. Repeat vigorously for 10 minutes. Form into a smooth ball, cover with waxed paper (oiled on one side), tucking paper under dough; cover loosely with towel. Let rest for *20 minutes.*

Prepare pans: oil bottom and sides. After 20 minutes, punch down dough with two doubled-up fists until it is like a large flat pancake. Cut exactly in half. Lift up one half at a time, fold over and seal ends. Flatten again with flat of hands into 8-inch circle.

Turn over two upper edges to form a triangular "hat," then roll in from each side to shape an 8-inch loaf, sealing in ends. Place in pans seam-side down. Turn on oven for 1 minute, then turn off. Place pans in center of oven, close door, let rise until dough is 1½–2 inches above pans (60 minutes–1½ hours).

Turn on oven to 350° F. (pans need not be removed from oven), bake for 35 minutes, or until loaf sounds hollow when thumped on bottom. (If it's a dull thud, return to pans, and bake 5–10 minutes longer.) Remove bread from pans immediately, cool on rack for 3–4 hours before slicing or freezing. Makes 2 small loaves. (For 3 large loaves, double all ingredients.)

100 Percent Whole-Wheat Bread

5½–6½ cups whole-wheat flour
2 teaspoons salt
¼ cup rolled wheat or triticale flakes
¼ cup buckwheat grains
2 packages active dry yeast

2 tablespoons molasses
1½ cups unsweetened apple juice
4 tablespoons margarine
2 8x4x2½-inch loaf pans, greased

In mixing bowl combine 1 cup *only* of the flour, salt, wheat flakes, buckwheat, and undissolved yeast. Mix well. Stir in molasses. Heat apple juice to quite hot; add margarine. Add to flour mixture and beat for 2 minutes. Stir in more flour, ½ cup at a time, until dough comes away from the bowl. Turn out on board. Cover with bowl. Let stand for 10 minutes.

Remove bowl; wash in cold water, then in hot water. When dry, grease bowl. Knead dough vigorously for 10 minutes until pliable and smooth. Place in bowl, turn to grease all over. Cover top of bowl with plastic wrap; warm oven for 1 minute, then turn off heat. Place dough in oven until doubled in volume (40–50 minutes). Test by pushing finger in dough; if imprint remains, it is ready.

Turn out dough onto floured surface and punch down. Cut in half; roll each half and shape into 8-inch length to fit pan. Place in pans seam-side down. Return to oven to rise until 1½ inches above pans. Bake at 375° F. for 35–40 minutes. When done, remove immediately and cool on rack for several hours. For a glossy crust, brush while hot with margarine. Makes 2 small loaves.

Herb Griffin's Seeded Whole-Wheat Bread

2¾–3 cups whole-wheat flour
1 package active dry yeast
2 tablespoons brown sugar or molasses
½ teaspoon salt
½ cup water

½ cup milk
2 tablespoons oil
1 egg
¼ cup wheat germ
½ cup sunflower kernels or sesame seeds

Place in mixing bowl 1¼ cups of the flour, the yeast, sugar, and salt. Beat to blend. Heat together the water, milk, and oil to a temperature of 120° F. (hot but not scalding). Add this mixture, the egg, wheat germ, and seeds to the flour-yeast mixture, beat to moisten (low speed on mixer), then beat vigorously or at medium speed for 3 minutes. Stir in remaining flour, enough to make a pliable dough which comes away from side of bowl and can be lifted in one piece. Knead about 5 minutes until smooth and elastic. Place in greased bowl, turning to grease all sides. Let rise until doubled in warm, protected place. Punch down and turn out; roll into loaf shape. Place in greased 8½x4x2½-inch pan. Let rise again until doubled, until dough is well above rim of pan. Bake in oven preheated to 375° F. for 35–40 minutes. Makes 1 loaf.

To make 2 loaves, double all ingredients. (If preferred, use ½ cup of wheat germ and only ¼ cup of sunflower or sesame seeds, in the 1-loaf recipe, and ½ cup each in the 2-loaf version.)

Fruited Oatmeal Bread

1 cup water	¾ cup lukewarm water
¾ cup milk	3 packages active dry yeast,
½ cup bran meal	or 2¾ tablespoons
2 teaspoons salt	1 cup oatmeal
6 tablespoons margarine	6½–7½ cups unbleached flour
⅓ cup honey	½ cup dried currants
¼ cup Kretchmer wheat germ	

Combine 1 cup of water and milk; bring almost to a boil. Stir in bran, salt, margarine, honey, and wheat germ. Pour ¾ cup of warm water in large mixing bowl; sprinkle in yeast and let stand for 3 minutes. Add bran mixture, oatmeal, and 1 cup flour (only). Beat vigorously for 2 minutes. Add currants and continue to add flour until dough comes away from sides of bowl, leaving bowl almost clean. Turn out on lightly floured surface, cover with a towel, let stand for 5 minutes.

Wash bowl; when dry, grease it. Knead dough vigorously for 10 minutes until pliable and smooth. Place in bowl; brush a little oil over top. Cover bowl with plastic wrap. Turn on oven for 1 minute; then turn it off. Place dough in an unlighted oven to rise until doubled, about 1 hour or until it passes finger-imprint test. Turn out on floured surface and punch down. Divide dough exactly in half; shape each into loaves to fit 8½x4x2½-inch pans. Again heat oven for 1 minute, then turn off heat and place pans in center of oven. Allow to rise until dough is 1½ inches above rim of pans. Turn on oven to 375° F. (it need not be preheated). Bake bread for 30 minutes, or until loaf sounds hollow on bottom when tapped. (If it makes a dull thud, return to pans and bake for 5–10 minutes longer.) For a glossy crust, brush tops with margarine while hot. Cool on racks for 3–4 hours. Makes 2 loaves.

Sour Rye Caraway Bread

2 packages active dry yeast
½ cup lukewarm water
¾ cup hot water
1 tablespoon salt
1 tablespoon molasses
2 tablespoons oil or shortening
1 cup unbleached all-purpose flour
1 cup buttermilk
3 cups dark rye flour
½ cup crushed brown rye Swedish crispbread
2 tablespoons caraway seeds
1½–2 cups whole-wheat flour

Dissolve yeast in lukewarm water in large mixing bowl. Combine hot water with salt, molasses, and oil or shortening; heat until quite hot, cool to lukewarm. Add to yeast.

Stir in white flour, then the buttermilk, then start adding rye flour mixed with the crushed crispbread, ½ cup at a time, beating until flour is completely moistened. Add caraway seeds and start adding whole-wheat flour ½ cup at a time until a soft, pliable dough is formed which can be picked up. Turn out onto lightly floured board. Cover; let rest for 10 minutes.

Knead until smooth, elastic, and blistered (at least 8 minutes). You may find it necessary to work in more whole-wheat flour. Oil or grease a 1-quart mixing bowl, heat it briefly, then put ball of dough in bowl, turning to grease on all sides. Cover bowl, put in warm place—but not too warm, because it should not rise too fast. When doubled in volume, test with finger. Punch down; let rise again (about 30 minutes). Divide into 2 parts. Shape each into a loaf and place in greased loaf pans; or shape each into a ball, higher in center, narrow around bottom, and place in lightly greased 8-inch cake pans. Let rise again until dough passes finger test. Preheat oven to 350° F. (moderate), bake bread about 50 minutes, or until bread sounds hollow when tapped. For glossy crust, brush top of loaves with melted butter or soft margarine. Turn out on rack, allow to cool. Makes 2 loaves.

Limpa
(Swedish Rye)

½ teaspoon baking soda
2 cups buttermilk
½ cup water
¼ cup dark molasses
1 tablespoon fennel seed
½ teaspoon crushed cardamom
½ tablespoon salt

3 tablespoons shortening or oil
1 package active dry yeast
½ cup crushed brown rye Swedish crispbread
2 cups unbleached flour
3–3½ cups dark rye flour
2 tablespoons melted butter

Add soda to buttermilk. In saucepan, combine water, molasses, fennel, cardamom, salt, and shortening. Bring just to a boil, remove from heat, and cool to lukewarm.

Add yeast to lukewarm mixture, stir to dissolve. Add soda-buttermilk mixture, crushed crispbread, and white flour; beat to make a smooth dough. Add rye flour, ½ cup at a time, beating until dough comes away from sides of bowl and can be lifted with wooden spoon in one piece. Turn out on lightly floured surface, knead until smooth and elastic. Place in greased heated bowl; cover. Set in warm, draft-free place and let rise until doubled (1½–2 hours). Punch down; knead again. Divide in half and make two round balls. Place on baking sheet and brush tops with melted butter. Let rise again until doubled (about 1 hour). Place in oven *preheated* to 375° F.; after 10 minutes, reduce heat to 350° F. Bake 35–45 minutes longer. Remove from oven and brush again with butter. Makes 2 loaves.

Whole-Wheat Dinner Rolls

½ cup warm water	2 teaspoons salt
2 packages active dry yeast	⅓ cup oil or soft shortening
1½ cups lukewarm milk	2 eggs
2 tablespoons brown sugar	3¾–4½ cups whole-wheat flour

Dissolve yeast in warm water in large mixing bowl. Combine milk, sugar, salt, and oil or shortening; heat until steaming. Combine in mixing bowl eggs, 2 cups of the flour, yeast, and milk mixture. Stir until flour is moistened. Continue to add flour, stirring, until dough becomes stiff; then add more flour until a smooth, pliable dough is formed that comes away from the sides of the bowl and can be lifted with spoon in one piece. Turn out onto floured board, let rest, covered with mixing bowl. Grease or oil a second bowl. (If these are to be refrigerator rolls or bread sticks, at this stage place in refrigerator—see *Refrigerator Rolls* below.)

If to be baked within 2 hours, let dough rise, covered, in a warm place until doubled (about 50 minutes). Punch down, and let rise again to approximately same volume. Then pinch off small pieces of dough and shape as desired, working in seeds or flavoring as suggested in following variations. Let rise once more, for about 20 minutes, or until dough passes finger test. Bake in preheated hot oven (400° F.) for 12–15 minutes until quite brown. Serve hot. Makes 1½–2 dozen, depending on size of rolls.

Refrigerator Rolls

Store ball of above dough, before kneading, in refrigerator for at least 2 hours or overnight. Remove about 2 hours before rolls are to be served. Let stand at room temperature for 30 minutes, then turn out onto floured board and knead for at least 5 minutes until very smooth and elastic. Pinch off pieces of dough and shape as desired, then let rise again until doubled, while preheating oven to 400° F. Bake 12–15 minutes for rolls, about 10 minutes for breadsticks. (See recipe variation, page 67.)

Sesame Seed Rolls

Work some sesame seeds into preceding dough as you knead. When dough has been shaped and *after* it has risen, brush with a mixture of 1 unbeaten egg white and 1 tablespoon of water, then sprinkle sesame seeds over top of each.

Buckwheat Cloverleaf Rolls

Work buckwheat grains into preceding dough as you shape it. Pinch off quite small pieces of dough, about the size of a nickel, and roll into balls between greased palms. Put three such small balls together in each muffin cup.

Wheat-Germ Parkerhouse Rolls

Pinch off pieces of dough the size of small eggs. Work into each some Kretchmer wheat germ, then press out into flat circles and fold over each halfway. Place small dab of butter on inside of each such roll. Moisten edges and press together. Bake as directed above.

Caraway-Seeded Rolls

Pinch off pieces of preceding dough the size of a small egg, work caraway seeds into dough, shape as desired. To form a twist or sailor's knot, pull and stretch dough to a long thin pencil shape, then form a knot. Brush outside with milk or melted butter before baking, as directed above. Serve warm (these get stale rather quickly).

Breadsticks

Pull out pieces of preceding dough the size of a walnut, stretch and pull, then roll on floured board below palms of hands until as thin as pencils. Scatter sesame seeds over the board as you roll, so some of seeds will be worked into the dough. Place on lightly greased or Teflon-coated baking sheet;

let rise until half again the original size, but not doubled. If thickly seeded sticks are wanted, brush tops with unbeaten egg blended with water, then sprinkle more seeds over sticks. Bake in preheated 400° F. oven for 8–10 minutes until well browned. Let cool until crisp and dry. If not to be served immediately, wrap in plastic. (These will be easier to handle if made as refrigerator rolls; see *Refrigerator Rolls,* page 66.)

Arabian Pocket Bread

2 packages active dry yeast	1 tablespoon bran meal
2 cups lukewarm water	1 teaspoon salt
2 cups unbleached all-purpose flour	3–4 cups whole-wheat flour
	3–4 tablespoons oil

Soften yeast in ¾ cup of lukewarm water. Place all-purpose flour, bran, salt, and 2 cups of the whole-wheat flour in a mixing bowl, forming a well in the center. Add yeast, remaining water, and 3 tablespoons of the oil to this "well," beating in flour until it is completely moistened. Knead until smooth and pliable, adding more whole-wheat flour as needed. Shape into 1 large ball and let stand in warm place until doubled (about 30 minutes). Turn out onto floured board, knead again until smooth and elastic, then divide into 16 equal pieces. Shape each piece into a ball, let rest for 1 hour at room temperature. Cut 16 squares of foil, each 7x7 inches, and place a ball on each square. Then with fingers, pat down the dough to form a circle no more than ½ inch thick. Brush remaining tablespoon of oil over the tops. Bake 2 at a time in an oven preheated to 450° F. (quite hot) for about 5 or 6 minutes, or until nicely browned. They will puff up as they bake, then fall with cooling to create a soft pocket in the center. When completely cold, slit so that pocket is opened. They can be used to hold a Sloppy Joe mixture, for sausages and cheese, hamburgers, or any sandwich filling, hot or cold. Makes 16. (They can be frozen after baking to be used as needed, or heated by slipping in toaster.)

Chapter 5

Appetizers
and Hors D'Oeuvres

The variety of salty snacks offered in every supermarket is stupendous—and frightening. Nine tenths of the snack foods qualify as "empty-calorie," made mostly of starch, chemicals, artificial flavors, artificial colors, salt, sugar, and fat. Among the few supermarket snack items that score high both for nutritional value and lack of sugar are Triscuits and certain of the rye crackers or wafers.

Fortunately there are many interesting and nutritious high-fiber snacks to be found in health stores. Yogurt chips, made with low-fat dehydrated yogurt, are excellent. There are both plain and "barbecue-flavored" sunflower kernels, brown rice chips, "wheat nuts," and imitation peanuts made of vegetable protein, besides, of course, dry-roasted nuts, Mexican pumpkin seeds, and toasted soybeans.

But there are many "fruits of Nature" that should be on the cocktail table. When chestnuts are available, roast them in the oven and serve hot as appetizers. (I was astonished to learn that chestnuts are low in fat—they taste quite the opposite.) Green and black olives, all the raw vegetable relishes, and cubes of avocado are also good sources of fiber.

Make your own whole-wheat Melba toast, and crackers, too. (There are two cracker recipes in Chapter 12.)

Cheese Balls

¼ cup crushed whole-bran cereal
¼ cup instant minced onion

1 8-ounce package Neufchâtel cheese, softened
½ cup salted peanuts, chopped fine or crushed

Work bran and onion into cheese by beating with spoon. Form 1-inch balls, rolling between palms of your hands. Refrigerate until firm, then roll in nuts, chill again until ready to serve. Makes about 25.

Sesame Cheese Balls

Omit the onion in the above recipe; roll the balls in toasted sesame seeds.

Caraway Cheese Balls

Instead of onion, add 2 tablespoons of caraway seeds to the cheese mixture and roll the cheese balls in minced parsley.

Wheat Chex Balls

Instead of onion, add very finely minced green pepper to the cheese mixture and roll the balls in crushed Wheat Chex.

Stuffed Celery

(LC)

24 2-inch pieces of celery
 1 8-ounce package Neufchâtel or farmers cheese, softened
 ½ cup chopped salted sunflower kernels

2 tablespoons whole-bran cereal
2 tablespoons chopped parsley or fresh coriander

Trim celery, selecting pieces suitable for stuffing. Combine remaining ingredients; place about 1 tablespoon of stuffing in each piece of celery. Makes about 1 cup stuffing.

Ham Roll-Ups

Using the preceding stuffing mixture, put a little inside thin-sliced ham, roll up, and secure with toothpicks.

Party Mix

1 cup Wheat Chex
1 cup spoon-size Shredded
  Wheat
1 cup Cheerios
1 tablespoon oil
1 teaspoon seasoned salt

¾ cup toasted soybeans or
  Spanish peanuts
¼–½ cup shelled pistachio nuts
½ cup raisins
½ cup chopped dried apricots

Put the three kinds of breakfast cereal in a skillet with oil; stir-fry until lightly toasted. (Do not burn!) Sprinkle while hot with seasoned salt. Place in bowl with remaining ingredients and mix well. The combination of sweet fruit and salty cereal and nuts is delightful. Keep stored on shelf in a covered container. Makes about 5 cups.

Oriental Nut Mix

2 tablespoons oil
¼ cup soy sauce
1 cup salted peanuts
½ cup blanched almonds

½ cup unsalted sunflower
  kernels
1 tablespoon celery seed
1 teaspoon sesame seed

Mix oil and soy sauce; add to nuts and sunflower kernels and spread out in a shallow pan. Sprinkle with celery and sesame seeds. Bake, stirring occasionally, in a 350° F. oven for about 20 minutes. Makes 2 cups.

Dips, Spreads, Pâtés

California Bran Dip

Make the famous California Dip using sour cream or plain yogurt with onion soup mix, but add to it ¼–⅓ cup of wheat germ or bran meal.

Yogurt Walnut Dip

¼ cup shelled walnuts
1 garlic clove, crushed
1 tablespoon olive oil
½ cup chopped radishes

1 cup plain yogurt
1 tablespoon whole-bran
  cereal or wheat germ
Salt and pepper to taste

Place walnuts in blender and beat until coarsely chopped; add remaining ingredients to blender in order given and beat to blend well. Makes about 1¼ cups. Serve as a dip for vegetable relishes.

Humus Dip

½ cup toasted sesame seeds
2 tablespoons olive oil
2 cups cooked or canned
  chickpeas

2 or 3 garlic cloves, crushed
Lemon juice to taste
Chopped parsley to taste

Place sesame seeds in blender with olive oil and beat until creamy. Drain chickpeas thoroughly, add to blender with crushed garlic, lemon juice, and a generous amount of parsley. Blend until mixture is very creamy. (In the Middle East, a little well is made in the center and olive oil is placed in the well.) Makes about 1¾ cups.

Guacamole

2 large ripe avocado
Juice of ½ lemon
1 tablespoon olive oil

1 tablespoon grated onion
Dash of Tabasco

Peel and stone avocados; chop, mash, and immediately sprinkle with lemon juice. Add remaining ingredients and keep in bowl tightly covered with plastic wrap until time to serve. Makes about 1½ cups. Serve as a dip.

Nutty Guacamole

Add to above mixture ½ cup of finely chopped sunflower "nuts" or pumpkin seeds.

Egg Nut Pâté

1 cup thinly sliced onion
3 tablespoons butter
¾ cup shelled walnuts, pecans, or hazelnuts

2 hard-cooked eggs
1 raw green chili pepper, seeded

Sauté onion in butter until quite soft. Place onions in blender with shelled nuts, eggs, and chili pepper. Beat just until well blended, not pureed. Makes 1½ cups. Delicious with whole-wheat crackers.

Cheese Nut Dip

¾–1 cup shredded or grated dried-up cheese
¼ cup salted peanuts, ground
2 tablespoons sunflower kernels, coarsely ground

½ cup creamed cottage cheese (small curd)
1–2 tablespoons milk
Dash of Tabasco

Use any bits and pieces of cheese you may have in the refrigerator, the more dried up the better. If quite hard, the cheese should be grated, if softer, put through a Mouli cheese shredder. The easiest way to grind peanuts is in a blender. Combine ingredients with just enough milk for creamy consistency. Skim milk may be used—or you may find you don't need milk at all. This mixture is good with carrot sticks especially, or may be served with celery cabbage cut into 2-inch lengths (and used as a scoop). Makes about 1½ cups.

Toasted Soybean Dip

1 cup toasted soybeans
1 garlic clove, or ½ teaspoon garlic powder
¼ cup minced parsley
2 tablespoons olive oil

2–3 tablespoons lemon juice
Salt to taste
2–3 tablespoons plain yogurt or sour cream

Crush soybeans in mortar with pestle, work in garlic—but use only a very small clove, or a small amount of garlic powder (the garlic flavor should be only a "suspicion"). Work in parsley, olive oil, lemon juice, and salt to make a thick paste. Thin with yogurt or sour cream. Very good with whole-wheat breadsticks. Makes 1¼ cups.

Hors D'Oeuvres

Celery Root Vinaigrette

(LC)

1 large celery root (celeriac)
Salt
Juice of ½ lemon
¼ cup olive oil or safflower
   oil

1 tablespoon vinegar
Several paper-thin onion
   slices, or ¼ cup thinly
   sliced scallion
1 teaspoon caraway seeds

Pare the brown outer rind of the celery root, cut root into slices, then into sticks or slivers, or grate coarsely. Sprinkle with salt and lemon juice immediately, then add oil, vinegar, and onion. Marinate at least 1 hour, tightly covered with plastic wrap. Makes about 2 cups, depending on the size of the celery root.

Turkish Cucumber Walnut Salad

(LC)

2 medium cucumbers
Salt, pepper to taste
1 teaspoon lemon juice
2 garlic cloves
1 tablespoon olive oil
1 tablespoon vinegar
¼ cup chopped walnuts

⅓ cup chopped green pepper
1 tablespoon chopped sweet
   red pepper
1 tablespoon chopped fresh
   mint, or ½ teaspoon dried
   mint, crushed

Partially peel cucumbers in strips, so that peel makes a striped effect. Slice, then chop. (The English cucumbers without seeds are preferable to the domestic variety for this dish.) Immediately sprinkle cucumber with salt, pepper, and lemon juice. Let stand ½ hour, then drain well (the salt makes the cucumbers "weep"). Crush garlic cloves in bowl, add olive oil and vinegar, then drained cucumbers, walnuts, the peppers, and mint. Marinate for 1 hour before serving. Makes 6 hors d'oeuvres servings.

Nutty Salade Russe

(LC)

1   10-ounce package frozen peas and carrots (or 1 cup cooked peas and diced cooked carrots)
¼   cup minced celery
2   tablespoons minced green pepper
2   tablespoons sunflower kernels

1   or 2 tablespoons whole-bran cereal
1   tablespoon olive oil
½   tablespoon vinegar or lemon juice
1–2 tablespoons mayonnaise
2   tablespoons chopped parsley
¼   teaspoon celery seeds
Salt, pepper to taste

Combine all ingredients; blend well. Serve chilled. Makes about 1½ cups of salad, to be served as part of an hors d'oeuvres assortment.

For better flavor, cook fresh peas and carrots separately, and marinate while still warm. Carrots, if cut in strips before cooking, can be sufficiently cooked for the salad in about 3 minutes.

Russian Herring Salad

(LC)

2   salt herrings
2   cups milk
1   medium onion, minced
1   tart, unpeeled red apple, chopped
2   slices Westphalian rye bread, in small pieces
½   teaspoon caraway seeds

2   tablespoons oil
2   tablespoons vinegar
6–8 small whole beets (cooked or canned), marinated
10–12 black olives
1   lemon, quartered
2   hard-cooked eggs, sliced

Soak herring in milk for 24 hours. Remove from milk (discard the milk). Bone and skin fish, and cut into small pieces or put through food grinder. Add onion, apple, rye bread, and caraway seeds. Blend thoroughly. Add oil and vinegar. Shape mixture into a mound on platter, surround with whole beets (which have been marinated separately in Oil-Vinegar Dressing), black olives and quartered lemon, and place egg slices over the top. Makes about 10 hors d'oeuvres servings.

Tabbouleh
(Lebanese Wheat Salad)

1 cup bulgur
Water
¾ cup lemon juice, or to
   taste
½–¾ cup olive oil
½ teaspoon salt, or to taste
1 cup minced onion
1 cup minced parsley

½ cup minced fresh mint, or
   1 tablespoon crushed dried
   mint
1 cup peeled tomato,
   chopped
1 cup minced celery
Crisp lettuce leaves or
   romaine

Add enough water to bulgur to cover; then squeeze out water, using your hands. Place moistened bulgur in bowl with lemon juice, oil, and salt. Stir to blend well. Add remaining ingredients (except lettuce), stir again. Cover and chill for 24 hours. Serve on a platter surrounded with small lettuce leaves. Each person is expected to scoop up bulgur with lettuce leaf, roll it up, and pop into the mouth. Makes 8–10 servings.

CHAPTER 6

Soups

The rediscovery of homemade soups is an integral part of the natural foods revolution. Soups that take hours to cook are a snap with a crock-pot and usually are hearty enough to become the main course at supper. Simple, low-calorie soups can be very quickly made in the Oriental manner, with thin slivers of raw vegetables added to a well-seasoned broth, cooked only a matter of minutes. These are excellent recipes for dieters.

Cold soups are chiefly of interest as a first course for a barbecue meal or for lunch in hot weather. Their great advantage is that they can be made up ahead and kept chilled, ready to serve whenever wanted. But all soups age graciously; most of them taste better the second time around.

Vegetable Soups

Japanese Pork and Vegetable Soup

(LC)

3 cups water
4 teaspoons beef stock concentrate
¼ cup very thin slivers of raw pork, carefully trimmed of fat

½ cup carrot slivers
¼ cup thinly sliced cauliflower buds
2 scallions, thinly sliced
1 teaspoon soy sauce
6 fresh spinach leaves, stems removed

Combine water, beef stock concentrate, and pork; bring to a boil, reduce heat, and cook 5–7 minutes. (As long as the pork is cut in such tiny pieces, this is time enough to cook

77

it completely.) Add carrots, cauliflower, and scallions, and cook 2–3 minutes. Add soy sauce and spinach. Serve at once—spinach should be merely limp, not cooked. Makes 4 servings.

Chinese Vegetable Soup

(LC)

2 cups clear chicken or
  beef broth
¼ cup thinly sliced carrots
¼ cup raw green beans in
  thin slivers

1 cup thin mushroom slices
1 tablespoon sliced scallion
8 sprigs watercress, chopped

Combine all ingredients but watercress; bring to a boil, cook for 2–3 minutes. Add watercress to hot soup and serve immediately. Makes 4 servings.

Quick Cream of Carrot Soup

(LC)

4 medium carrots, scraped,
  thinly sliced or diced
1 tablespoon minced onion
  or scallion
1 stalk celery, minced*
1 tablespoon minced celery
  leaves
2 tablespoons butter

1 tablespoon soy flour
1 cup water
1 teaspoon salt
2 cups milk
1 tablespoon crushed
  peanuts
2 tablespoons minced parsley

Cook carrots, onion, and celery in butter over low to medium heat, stirring frequently (about 3 minutes). Add flour and blend with vegetables. Slowly add water and salt; cook covered for 5 minutes over low heat. Uncover, add milk and peanuts, and cook just until milk is heated through. Serve topped with parsley. Makes 4 servings.

*Discard all or most of leaves.

Curried Green Pea Soup

2 cups cooked or canned
   tiny green peas
1½ cups vegetable broth or
   liquid from peas
¼–½ teaspoon curry powder
1 teaspoon instant minced
   onion

Salt to taste
1 cup homogenized milk
2 tablespoons sour cream
Minced chives or parsley
Sautéed Wheat Chex
   (for croutons)

Puree cooked peas with the broth in blender, or force through food mill. Season with curry powder, onion, and salt (if needed). Bring just to a boil, turn off heat, and stir in milk. Top each serving with sour cream, parsley or chives, and croutons. Makes 4 servings.

Tomato Avocado Soup

2 10½-ounce cans condensed
   tomato soup
2 soup cans water
1 large ripe avocado
1 small garlic clove,
   crushed, or dash of
   garlic powder

Dash of Tabasco or cayenne
2 tablespoons sour cream
Chopped pumpkin seeds

Combine soup and water, add chunks of peeled avocado, garlic, and Tabasco or cayenne. Beat in blender until smooth. Serve topped with sour cream and the chopped seeds. Makes 5 or 6 servings.

For a hot soup, do not puree avocado but serve thin slices of it floating in the hot soup, top with sour cream.

Portuguese Watercress Soup

2 medium potatoes, peeled,
   diced
1 small white onion,
   quartered
5 cups water

1 teaspoon salt, or to taste
1 bunch watercress, stems
   removed
1 cup small croutons

Cook potatoes and onion in salted water until quite soft, then force liquid and vegetables through food mill so that liquid is a thin gruel. Add water if necessary to replace any lost through evaporation. Break watercress into pieces. Stir-fry croutons (cut from oatmeal or whole-wheat bread) until lightly browned; drain on absorbent paper. Just before serving, reheat the potato gruel, add watercress, cook just until limp. Serve topped with croutons. Makes 6 servings.

Portuguese Spinach Soup

Follow the recipe above, but use ½ pound of loose fresh spinach leaves (chopped) instead of watercress and cook about 2 minutes.

Caldo Verde

4 medium potatoes, peeled, diced
2 onions, peeled, quartered
8 cups water
2 teaspoons salt, or to taste
2 tablespoons oil
1 cup collard greens shredded as fine as grass blades
Diced ham, sliced chorizo sausage, or linguine sausage

Make a gruel by cooking potatoes and onions in salted water until very soft, then force through food mill. Replace in kettle, add collard greens and ham or sausage. Cook about 10 minutes, or until greens are tender. This is a popular national dish of Portugal. Makes 8–10 servings.

Russian Borscht

2½ quarts (10 cups) water
2 tablespoons salt
8 peppercorns
2 pounds soup meat with bone (hind shank of beef)
2 large carrots, scraped, sliced
1 cup chopped celeriac or celery
2 onions, sliced
2 tablespoons butter or oil
2 bunches beets with greens
1 tablespoon vinegar
4 cups shredded white or green cabbage
2 cups canned tomatoes for cooking
Sour cream

This, the authentic borscht of Russia, is a meal in itself. One should start the preparation a day ahead. Put water, salt, peppercorns, and meat with bone in kettle and bring to a boil. Simmer gently for 2 hours, skimming occasionally, until meat is very tender. Remove meat; separate meat from bones, cut meat into fine pieces, and reserve.

Clarify broth by pouring through fine cheesecloth into a deep bowl. Chill. When cold, fat will have solidified on top and is easy to remove.

The next step, the following day, is to sauté carrots, celeriac (or celery), and onions in butter until soft, stirring often (about 5 minutes). Do not allow to brown. Remove the leaves from beets and chop fine. Put these aside. Cut raw beet roots into slivers. Then assemble soup: into a big soup kettle place the carrot mixture, beet greens, chopped beets, meat, vinegar, cabbage, and tomatoes, and the clarified broth. Bring to a boil, and cook for 15 minutes. Taste and adjust seasonings. Serve topped with sour cream and accompanied by dark rye bread and butter. Makes 12–15 servings.

Vegetarian Borscht

Instead of making broth with meat, use vegetable or onion bouillon cubes and water, adding all the vegetables listed above. Instead of serving the bread separately, slightly stale rye bread may be broken into the soup and cooked with the vegetables, so that it thickens the broth.

Cold Soups

Chilled Cream of Pumpkin Soup

4 cups chicken broth	1 cup whole milk
¼ cup onion, minced	½ ripe avocado, thinly sliced
3 scallions, chopped	¼ cup heavy cream, whipped,
2 cups cooked or canned	or sour cream
pumpkin (1-pound can)	Sunflower or pumpkin seeds
Salt to taste	

Combine broth, onion, and scallions and simmer for 15 minutes. Add pumpkin and salt, blend well, and simmer for 5 minutes after mixture again comes to a boil. Puree in blender until smooth. When cool, add milk. Chill thoroughly. Serve in cups or bowls with thin slices of avocado on each, and decorate each with dollops of whipped or sour cream topped with chopped sunflower or pumpkin seeds. Makes 6–8 servings.

Senegalese Soup

2 cans condensed cream of
  chicken soup
1½ cups milk
1 teaspoon curry powder
1 cup plain yogurt or sour
  cream

1 egg yolk
½ cup chopped peanuts
½ cup shredded coconut
½ cup paper-thin slices of
  unpeeled cucumber

Combine soup, milk, and curry powder; slowly stir in yogurt. Heat, stirring constantly, until quite hot—but do not allow to boil. Beat egg yolk until thick; add to it a little hot soup at a time, beating until thickened. Chill soup. Serve cold, passing peanuts, coconut, and cucumber as garnish. Makes 6 servings.

Chilled Fruit Soup

½ cup dried apricots
½ cup raisins
½ cup pitted prunes
2 or 3 dried pears or
  peaches (optional)
8 cups water
2 fresh peaches or pears,
  peeled, sliced thin

2 apples, cored but not
  peeled, chopped
1 cup fresh blackberries or
  blueberries
2 tablespoons lemon juice
Honey to taste, if needed

Combine dried fruits, cover with water, bring to a boil, and simmer over low heat for about 30 minutes. Add fresh fruits and cook for 3–5 minutes longer. Remove from heat and add lemon juice. Cool to room temperature; add honey if needed. Chill. Serve cold with a dollop of honey-flavored yogurt on each serving. This has a winey flavor although it contains no wine. It is a lovely summer luncheon dish, and nothing else is needed to complete the meal but cheese and bread. Makes 8 servings.

Soups Made with Beans and Other Legumes

Every country has its special bean soups, and they are always hearty, filling dishes that can be served as a main course, or as first course followed by a light meal. (For more about cooking legumes, see page 164.)

Soybean Supper Soup

1 cup green (dried) soybeans
1 teaspoon salt
Cold water
2 medium onions, quartered
1 can condensed tomato
  soup
2 large carrots, scraped
  and diced
½ cup red (pink) lentils
1 tablespoon chopped fresh
  coriander or parsley
1 cup green beans, broken in
  pieces, or 1 cup shelled or
  frozen green peas
1 cup chopped collard or
  turnip greens, fresh or
  frozen
1 cup whole-wheat croutons
  or Wheat Chex, sautéed in
  oil until crisp

This is a good candidate for crock-pot cookery because it requires very long, slow cooking. Place beans in water to cover at least an inch above the beans and soak overnight. Or place beans and water in crock-pot or in oven casserole (covered) and cook overnight at 200°. Next day add more water, again covering the beans by at least an inch. Add onions and canned tomato soup. Simmer at lowest heat for 2½–3 hours, or until beans are almost tender. Add additional liquid if necessary; taste for seasoning.

Add carrots, lentils, fresh coriander or parsley, and green beans or peas. Cook for 20 minutes; add collard or turnip greens, and cook 10–15 minutes longer, or until all ingredients are tender. Serve in soup plates topped with croutons. Makes about 6 servings.

Note: Be sure to use *red* lentils; *brown* lentils would require much longer cooking. Millet grains may be added instead of red lentils.

Middle Eastern Lentil Soup

2 cups brown lentils
2 medium onions, cut in sticks
2 or 3 garlic cloves, slit
¼ cup chopped fresh coriander, or 1 tablespoon dried cilantro
½ teaspoon thyme
2 quarts water (or more)

2 teaspoons salt
¼ teaspoon black pepper
½ cup converted long-grain rice
Juice of ½ lemon, or 1 tablespoon vinegar
Whole-wheat croutons, sautéed in olive oil

Wash and pick over lentils (they need not be soaked). Sauté onion, garlic, and coriander in oil. Combine with lentils and add thyme, water, salt, and pepper. Bring to a boil, then simmer gently tightly covered for 1–2 hours, or until lentils are soft. Add more water as needed. During last half hour, add rice. Sprinkle with lemon juice or vinegar just before serving. Serve topped with croutons. Makes about 8 servings.

Portuguese Kidney Bean Soup

½ pound dried red kidney beans, soaked overnight and drained
2 quarts cold water
1 onion, quartered
2–3 teaspoons salt

¼ cup uncooked converted rice
1 cup finely chopped collard greens
Seasonings to taste
Dash of vinegar

Cover presoaked beans with water; add onion and salt. Cook, covered, over low heat until tender (about 2 hours). Beat in blender to puree, or force through food mill. Add rice, bring to a boil, reduce heat, and cook for 10 minutes. Add collard greens and continue to cook until greens are tender. Adjust seasonings; add vinegar. Simple as this sounds, it makes a most delicious soup. Makes 6–8 servings.

Shortcut version: Use two 1-pound cans kidney beans with the liquid; puree in blender and add more water to bring to desired consistency. Heat, add chopped or instant minced onion, rice, and collard greens and cook until greens are tender and rice soft. Add vinegar last.

Minestrone

1 cup (½ pound) dried large white beans
1 large onion, sliced
1 garlic clove, crushed
2 celery stalks, chopped, with some of leaves
2 tablespoons chopped parsley
1 large carrot, scraped and diced
½ cup whole-wheat macaroni shells (from health store)

¼ cup olive oil
1 or 2 small white turnips, or 1 large parsnip, peeled and diced
1 can (1 pound) plum tomatoes
1 cup finely chopped kale or collard greens
Grated Parmesan cheese

Soak beans in water to cover overnight; drain. Add fresh water (2 quarts) and salt; bring to a boil, then simmer gently for 1½–2 hours, or until tender. Separately sauté onion, garlic, celery, carrots, and parsley in oil until soft, turning frequently to avoid scorching. Add this mixture to beans with remaining ingredients. Cook until vegetables are tender and macaroni shells are *al dente*. Makes 8–10 hearty servings.

Yankee Bean Soup

1 pound (2 cups) navy beans
3 quarts (12 cups) water
2–3 teaspoons salt
1 ham hock or ham bone
1 medium onion, sliced

1 celery stalk with leaves, chopped
¼ teaspoon thyme
1 cup canned tomatoes for cooking

Soak beans overnight; drain, add fresh water and salt and remaining ingredients. Cook 2–3 hours; remove ham hock, chop meat into small pieces, return meat to soup. Do not puree. Serve topped with minced parsley. Makes 10–12 hearty servings.

Black Bean Soup

2 cups (1 pound) dried
  black beans
2 teaspoons salt
2–3 quarts cold water
1 small onion, sliced
2 celery stalks with leaves,
  chopped

2 tablespoons butter
¼ teaspoon prepared mustard
Pinch of cayenne pepper
1 lemon, thinly sliced
2 hard-cooked eggs, chopped

Soak beans overnight and drain. Add 2 quarts of cold water and salt and bring to a boil. Sauté onion and celery in butter for about 2 minutes; add to beans with mustard. Cook covered over lowest heat for 2–3 hours until beans are very soft. Keep an eye on the kettle and add more water from time to time as necessary (unless cooking beans in a crock-pot). Puree the mixture in a blender, add cayenne and any other seasoning desired. Reheat, adding the lemon slices. Serve topped with chopped egg, with lemon slices floating in soup. Makes about 10 servings. Leftovers may be frozen for later use.

Note: Black beans require longer cooking than most other legumes; if possible, use a pressure cooker for this soup.

Succotash Chowder

¼ pound salt pork, cubed,
  or ¼ cup oil or butter
1 large onion, chopped
2 medium potatoes, peeled
  and diced
1 green pepper, seeded and
  diced
1½ cups corn kernels scraped
  from cob, or 1 12-ounce
  can kernel corn, drained

2 teaspoons salt, or to taste
Freshly ground black
  pepper
⅛ teaspoon celery salt
Pinch of cayenne
1 10-ounce package frozen
  baby limas, thawed
¼ teaspoon paprika
1 quart milk
Health bread croutons

Draw out fat from salt pork in heavy skillet; remove and save the crisply browned chunks for garnish. Sauté onion and potatoes until golden in the drawn-out pork fat. Add green pepper, corn, salt, and other seasonings including paprika; stir and cook for 1 minute. Add limas and milk. Cook uncovered over very low heat (do not allow to boil) until vegetables are tender (about 15 minutes). Serve topped with croutons and reserved salt pork cubes. Makes about 8 servings.

(For a vegetarian soup, omit salt pork and use butter or margarine.)

Cream of Lima Bean Soup

1 cup dried lima beans
6–8 cups cold water
1½ teaspoons salt, or to taste
¼ cup chopped onion
¼ cup chopped carrot
2 tablespoons butter or
  margarine
1 tablespoon chopped fresh
  dill, or 1 teaspoon dill
  weed

Dash cayenne or powdered
  ginger
1 tablespoon whole-wheat
  flour
1 cup whole milk
Whole-wheat croutons, or
  Wheat Chex

Soak beans overnight; drain. Add 6 cups of cold water and salt. Simmer until beans are soft (about 2 hours). Add more water if necessary during cooking. Puree in blender or force through food mill. Sauté onion and carrot in butter or margarine until golden and soft, but not browned. Add dill, cayenne or ginger, stir in flour, allow to bubble a few seconds, then slowly stir in milk. Add the pureed beans, and any other seasonings to taste. Heat through. Serve topped with croutons. Makes 8–10 servings.

Mexican Chicken Avocado Soup

½ cup dried pinto beans
4 cups water
1 cup tomato juice
2 teaspoons salt
2 chicken legs
1 onion, chopped
¼ teaspoon oregano

¼ teaspoon dried basil
1 small carrot, thinly sliced
½ cup green beans, cut in
  small pieces
Dash of Tabasco
½ ripe avocado, cut in small
  pieces

Soak beans overnight; drain. Add to 4-quart heavy saucepan or crock-pot with water, tomato juice, and salt. Cook covered at lowest heat for 2 hours; add more water if necessary. Remove beans with slotted spoon, mash, return to kettle with chicken legs, onion, and herbs. Cook for 1 hour longer; remove chicken, discard skin and bones, return minced chicken meat to kettle. Add vegetables; cook for 10 minutes longer. Add Tabasco and avocado and cook for 2–3 minutes longer. Makes about 10 servings.

Lentil Soup Catalan

Remnants of baked ham with bone	2 cups brown lentils
1 large or 2 small onions, sliced	3 quarts water
	1½ teaspoons salt
2 or 3 garlic cloves, minced	½ teaspoon marjoram
	Whole-wheat French bread
3 tablespoons shortening	½ cup coarsely grated Swiss cheese

Brown onion and garlic in fat in large heavy kettle or crock-pot. Add lentils (they do not need presoaking), water, and seasonings. Add ham bone with any bits of leftover meat. Cover. Simmer over lowest heat until lentils are very tender (about 2 hours).

To serve, cut bread in thick pieces, place 1 or 2 pieces in bottom of each soup bowl, sprinkle Swiss cheese over bread, then ladle in the hot soup. Cheese will melt from the heat of the soup. Makes 8 or more servings.

Other Soups

Oxtail Soup

(LC)

2 pounds oxtail, cut in pieces
1 quart water
1 garlic clove, chopped
4 small onions, peeled
1 can (1 pound) tomatoes
1 teaspoon salt, or to taste
¼ teaspoon thyme
¼ teaspoon dill weed or crushed fennel
2 tablespoons sherry (optional)
4 carrots, scraped and diced
1 cup sliced celeriac or celery
1 cup cut green beans or limas
1 cup sliced okra, fresh or frozen
Whole-wheat croutons

Wash meat, pat dry, place in shallow pan, and bake uncovered in hot oven (preheated to 450° F.) until nicely browned, turning once. Or brown in heavy skillet. Transfer to large kettle. Pour off fat from pan; deglaze browned bits with hot water and add to kettle. Add water, garlic, onions, canned tomatoes, salt, and herbs. Simmer covered for 2–3 hours, or until meat is very tender. Skim broth occasionally. Add more water as needed. Add carrots, celeriac (or celery), and beans when meat seems tender; cook for 10 minutes. If sherry is used, add now. Add okra and cook about 3 minutes longer (okra should still be bright green and a little crisp). Serve with croutons as garnish. This is a hearty supper soup, needing only a big salad and a fruit dessert. Serves 6–8.

Polish Bread Soup

3 cups stale cubes of whole-grain rye bread (or use any health bread plus broken brown rye Swedish crisp-bread)
2 tablespoons meat drippings or butter
2 medium onions, chopped
2 medium carrots, scraped and chopped
1 leek, white part only, chopped
½ cup green beans, broken in small pieces
1 celery stalk, diced
1 parsnip, peeled and diced
6 cups water
Salt to taste
½ cup sour cream

Put 2 cups of bread cubes (or bread and broken crispbread) in a bowl, cover with hot water, and let stand until soft; then squeeze out and discard water. Sauté remaining bread (cut in small cubes) in drippings or butter until browned; set aside to use as croutons.

Combine water-softened bread with vegetables, water, and salt; bring to a boil and simmer about 40 minutes. Serve topped with sour cream and croutons. Makes 8 servings.

Sopa Castilla La Vieja
(Soup of Old Castile)

6 cups beef consommé
2 tablespoons oil
⅓ cup crushed almonds
2 cups toasted or sautéed whole-wheat croutons
½ cup toasted almond slivers
¼ cup grated Parmesan cheese

Heat consommé. Make a paste by working the oil into the crushed almonds with a wooden pestle. Stir paste into the hot consommé, blending well. Adjust seasonings.

Pour soup into 6 heatproof earthenware bowls; top each with some of the croutons and some of the cheese. Place under broiler until cheese is lightly browned. Remove and sprinkle slivered almonds over the top. Makes 8 servings.

CHAPTER 7

Adding Fiber to Meat,
Fish, and Poultry

While dietary fiber is found only in plant foods, it's easy to add it to entrees of animal protein. For stuffings, thickeners, extenders, and breading, use whole-grain breads and cereals and add vegetables, fruits, nuts, seeds, and legumes to entrees of meat, fish, and fowl. A beef stew with vegetables, for example, can be a good fiber source—depending on the vegetables.

In addition to the entrees in this chapter, others will be found in Chapters 8 and 9.

Hamburgers, Meatballs, and Meatloaves

Use bran as an extender to make plumper, juicier hamburgers and bigger meatballs. It's economical and a good health practice.

In recipes that call for an egg, people on cholesterol diets may use 1 tablespoon of soy flour as a binder instead—or simply use the white of the egg (only the yolk contains cholesterol).

Instead of catsup, why not use Dijon or Chinese mustard as a condiment? Catsup is high in sugar, and when hamburgers are drowned in it, that's a lot of unnecessary sucrose and calories. (Of course, if only a tablespoon of catsup is added to a recipe for 6–8 patties, the amount is negligible.)

Many prepared mustards contain some sugar, but the Dijon style does not. You can prepare your own by thinning powdered mustard with water or white wine.

Juicy Economy Hamburgers

2 pounds extra-lean ground
  beef
1 cup whole-wheat bread,
  broken in pieces

1 tablespoon pure bran meal
½ cup milk
2 teaspoons salt
1 tablespoon catsup

Soak bread and bran in milk until very soft. Add to meat
with salt and catsup and work with fingers until well blended
but not compact. Shape into patties. Broil or pan-broil to
medium (not rare). Makes 10.

Hi-Fiber Hamburgers

1 pound ground chuck
⅓ cup finely crushed
  Shredded Wheat
1 tablespoon bran meal
1 egg, beaten

1 teaspoon catsup
1 teaspoon salt
½ teaspoon horseradish or
  Dijon mustard (optional)

Combine all ingredients and work lightly with fingers to blend
well; shape into patties. Broil or pan-broil to desired doneness.
Makes 6.

Nutty Hamburgers

1½ pounds lean ground beef
1 egg
⅓ cup finely crushed
  Shredded Wheat or
  Wheat Chex
½ cup coarsely crushed peanuts or toasted soybeans

1 tablespoon instant minced
  onion (optional)
1 tablespoon wheat germ
  or bran meal
1½ teaspoons salt

Combine all ingredients; knead lightly and shape into plump
patties. Pan-fry in just enough oil to moisten bottom of pan.
Makes 8.

Lamb Meatballs with Tomato Sauce

MEATBALLS:
- 1 pound lamb patties*
- 1 cup crushed Triscuits
- ¼ cup chopped sunflower seeds
- ¾ teaspoon salt
- 1 small-to-medium egg
- ⅓ cup water or tomato juice

SAUCE:
- 1 cup tomato sauce, or 1 8-ounce can
- ½ cup dry white wine or orange juice
- Pinch of thyme or oregano
- Salt, pepper

To make meatballs, combine all ingredients, knead to mix well, then form into 1½-inch balls. Sauté in pan barely moistened with fat or oil to prevent sticking, or sprinkle salt over heated pan. Move meatballs before they have browned to prevent sticking (or use a Teflon-coated pan). Cook until well browned on all sides. Remove from pan; pour off all fat.

To the pan drippings, that is, the bits of brown sticking to the pan (what the French call the "glaze"), add the tomato sauce, wine or juice, and seasonings. Simmer, stirring, until sauce is reduced. Replace meatballs in sauce and simmer over low heat for 10–15 minutes, turning several times. Makes 4 or 5 servings.

*If preferred, ground beef may be used instead of lamb.

Swedish Meatballs

- 1 pound ground meatloaf mixture (beef, veal, and pork)
- 2 eggs
- 1 teaspoon salt
- Pinch of nutmeg
- 1 slice whole-grain bread, wheat or rye

- ½ cup milk
- 1 tablespoon minced onion or parsley
- 3 cups beef or chicken broth
- 1½ tablespoons whole-wheat or soy flour
- ½ cup sour cream

Combine meatloaf mixture, eggs, salt, and nutmeg. Break bread into pieces and soak in milk until soft. Add to meat mixture along with onion or parsley. Knead until well blended; form into 1-inch balls.

Heat broth to boiling. Add meatballs to simmering (not boiling) broth but avoid crowding pan. Cook meatballs about 15 minutes, or until they rise to top of liquid. Remove with slotted spoon; add more until all are cooked. Thicken broth by adding a little broth to the flour, stir until smooth, then slowly add remaining broth. Return to heat and cook, stirring with whisk, until thickened and smooth. Remove from heat, cool slightly, then stir in sour cream. Pour sauce over meatballs. Keep warm in covered casserole in 300° oven until time to serve. Makes 4–6 servings.

My Family's Favorite Meatloaf

1 pound extra-lean ground beef	¼ cup tomato catsup
1 pound ground lean pork	2 teaspoons salt
2 eggs	1 tablespoon lemon juice
1 teaspoon grated lemon rind	½ cup milk or water
1 cup finely crushed Shredded Wheat or Triscuits	1 small onion, minced
	1 tablespoon minced parsley
	1 tablespoon oil

Combine all ingredients but oil; knead to blend well. Place meat in greased shallow roasting pan and form into loaf shape. Brush oil over top. Bake in moderate (350° F.) oven for 1½ hours. When crisply brown on outside, carefully remove from pan with spatula and allow to stand at room temperature for 15 minutes before slicing. Makes about 10 thick slices.

To make gravy: Pour off excess fat from pan, reserving about 2 tablespoons of pan drippings, including the brown part. Stir in 2 tablespoons of whole-wheat or soy flour, 1 teaspoon of catsup, and about ¼ teaspoon of salt; then slowly add 1 cup of water. Simmer about 5 minutes. Turn off heat. Stir in 2 tablespoons of sour cream or plain yogurt. Adjust seasonings to taste. (Only whole-milk yogurt, such as Dannon's, can be used successfully in making gravies or sauces. Low-fat yogurt thickened with gelatin and vegetable gum simply does not work as well nor give the same flavor.)

Tangy Meatloaf

¼ cup tomato paste
½ teaspoon dry mustard, or 1 teaspoon Dijon mustard
2 teaspoons Worcestershire sauce
1 tablespoon instant minced onion
2 tablespoons minced green pepper

1½–2 teaspoons seasoned salt
¼ teaspoon black pepper
1 teaspoon chili powder
1 egg
1½ cups Wheat Chex crushed to ¾ cup
1½ pounds extra-lean ground beef

In a large bowl combine tomato paste and mustard; remove half the mixture to a small bowl to reserve for topping.

To remaining mixture in bowl, add Worcestershire, onion, green pepper, salt, black pepper, chili powder, and egg. Blend well. Stir in crushed cereal and ground beef, blending thoroughly. Shape into a loaf and place in shallow roasting pan. Bake at 350° F. (moderate oven) for 65 minutes. Remove from oven, moisten reserved tomato paste mixture with just enough water to make it easier to spread, then brush over top of meatloaf. Return to oven and bake for 15 minutes longer. Makes 6 servings.

Ham Loaf with Horseradish Sauce

5 cups cooked ham, put through grinder
¼ cup rolled oats (or rye flakes or triticale flakes)
2 tablespoons All Bran
1 tablespoon buckwheat grains

1 cup milk
½ teaspoon salt
1 tablespoon Worcestershire or soy sauce
2 eggs

Soften oats (or other cereal flakes), bran, and buckwheat in milk while grinding the ham. Combine all ingredients, blend well, and shape into a loaf. Place in lightly greased loaf pan. Bake in oven preheated to 350° F. (moderate) for 1 hour.

Let stand at room temperature for 5–10 minutes before slicing. Serve with Horseradish Sauce. Makes 8 servings.

Horseradish Sauce

Blend together 1 cup of sour cream or (to cut calories) plain yogurt and 1–2 tablespoons of grated horseradish.

Stews, Roasts, and Cutlets

Sweet and Sour Beef Stew

(LC)

1½ pounds boneless beef for stew, cut in cubes
1 tablespoon oil
1 slice whole-wheat bread, fried in 1 tablespoon olive oil
1 large or 2 medium onions, thickly sliced, chopped
1 garlic clove, slit
¼ cup tomato sauce
½ cup water
2 tablespoons vinegar or lemon juice
8 pitted prunes, chopped
½ green pepper, cut in pieces
1 small (4–5 inch) yellow squash, thickly sliced
3 tablespoons chopped parsley
2 tablespoons shredded coconut

In heavy pot, sauté meat in oil until browned on all sides. Fry the bread separately in olive oil on both sides. (This may sound strange, but it gives the bread, and the sauce of the stew, special smoothness.) Remove bread, drain on absorbent paper, then cut into squares.

Add onion and garlic to pot with meat; let cook until garlic is lightly browned and soft, then crush garlic with tines of fork. Add tomato sauce, water, and vinegar or lemon juice. Simmer, covered, for 1 hour. Then add prunes, green pepper, squash, and the fried bread. Cook *uncovered* for ½ hour longer. Serve topped with chopped parsley and coconut. Delicious and unusual! Makes 4 or 5 servings.

Lamb with Beans, Greek Style

1 pound dried white beans
(Great Northern or
marrow beans)
1 pound boneless lean lamb
from shoulder
2 tablespoons olive oil
2 onions, chopped
1 or 2 garlic cloves, crushed

½ cup canned tomatoes for
cooking
2 teaspoons salt
4–6 cups water
¼ cup minced parsley or
fresh coriander
½ teaspoon thyme

Soak beans overnight; drain. Add boiling water to beans, let stand for 5 minutes, drain again. Brown meat in oil in large casserole, Dutch oven, or crock-pot. Add onions and garlic; cook 2 or 3 minutes. Add remaining ingredients. Simmer, covered, about 3 hours, adding more water as needed. Makes 8–10 servings.

Fruit-Stuffed Veal or Lamb Shoulder

1 veal or lamb shoulder or
breast, boned and trimmed
for stuffing
1 small onion, chopped
1 green or red sweet pepper,
chopped
1 small garlic clove, crushed
2 tablespoons butter or
margarine
1 cup dried apricots,
chopped

1 cup bran meal
2 slices stale whole-grain
bread, broken in small
pieces
½ teaspoon salt
¼ teaspoon thyme
Oil or melted butter
Salt to taste
½ cup red wine or tomato
juice

Lay boned meat out flat; trim edges to make a uniform shape and mince the trimmings to use in the stuffing. (Or, if you have a friendly butcher, ask him to cut a pocket for you.) Sauté onion, green pepper, and garlic in butter until lightly browned and soft. Add to minced meat with apricots, bran, bread, salt, and thyme. Blend well; spread mixture over meat (or push inside if it has a pocket for stuffing). Roll up, tie with cord as you would a parcel for mailing. Brush outside of meat with oil or butter, sprinkle with salt. Place in shallow roasting pan and roast at 300° F. (slow oven) for 3½ hours, or until a meat thermometer registers 170° F. Baste occasionally with wine (or tomato juice). When done, let stand at room temperature about 10 minutes before slicing. In the meantime, make gravy with pan drippings, if desired. Makes 6–8 servings.

Chicken, Turkey, Duck, Cornish Hens

The most obvious way to add fiber to poultry is in bread stuffing, but there are other delicious ways—with fruit, coconut, nuts, and, of course, vegetables.

As suggested several times before, "breading" need not be done with breadcrumbs. Crushed breakfast cereals and crushed rolled oats, rye flakes, or crushed wheat berries can be used. And for dumplings or pastry crusts, whole-wheat flour may be used rather than white flour; or use white flour but add bran.

The following recipe for Fruit-Stuffed Chicken has first place in this section because when I served it to friends not long ago, they all asked for the recipe.

Fruit-Stuffed Chicken

(LC)

1 roasting chicken, 4–5 pounds
½ lemon
1 small onion, coarsely chopped
1–2 tablespoons chopped parsley
2 tablespoons oil or margarine
½ cup chopped pitted prunes
¼ cup toasted soybeans
1 cup chopped apple (not peeled)
⅛ teaspoon slivered chopped ginger root (optional)
Few thin slices lemon peel, chopped
2–3 slices stale whole-wheat bread, diced
Salt, pepper to taste

Prepare chicken for roasting: cut away all visible portions of fat, rub outside skin all over with the cut side of a lemon, then sprinkle inside and out with salt. Put wings behind the neck.

Combine in a bowl, in order given, all the remaining stuffing ingredients. Mix well. Place inside breast cavity of chicken, then truss the opening. Tie legs together, if desired. Roast in a moderate (350° F.) oven for 1–1½ hours until leg moves easily and skin of chicken is a glossy golden brown. Let stand at room temperature for at least 15 minutes for easier carving, while preparing gravy. Makes 4–6 servings.

To make gravy: Pour off excess fat, keeping about 2–3 tablespoons of drippings in pan. Stir in an equal amount of whole-wheat or soy flour, stirring over low heat until well blended. Slowly add 1–1¼ cups of chicken broth (made with neck and giblets while the chicken was roasting). Salt to taste. Simmer until smooth and slightly thickened.

For turkey stuffing: Triple all stuffing ingredients for a 12-pound turkey.

Rye-Flaked Oven-Fried Chicken
(LC)

This will give the old oven-fried chicken quite a different new flavor. Use rye flakes instead of flour or a bake-and-shake commercial mix. Crush the flakes in a blender or with a rolling pin, mix with salt and pepper, place in a brown paper bag, then shake a few chicken pieces at a time in the mixture.

Melt 2 or 3 tablespoons of butter, margarine, or vegetable shortening in a shallow roasting pan; place the chicken pieces in the melted fat, bake in a moderately hot (375–400° F.) oven for 15–20 minutes; turn each piece, continue baking until crisp and brown on all sides.

If gravy is desired, pour off excess fat, keeping only the browned essence, and stir just enough soy flour into this to absorb the fat. Slowly add liquid (chicken broth or water), cook and stir over moderate heat until thickened and smooth. Add salt to taste.

(Rolled oats may be used instead of rye flakes. These are softer than rye flakes but become crisp with baking.)

Chicken Amandine

(LC)

1 broiler-fryer, cut up
1 cup chicken broth
¼ cup whole-wheat flour
1 teaspoon salt
4 tablespoons clarified butter, or 2 tablespoons each butter and oil

½ cup slivered blanched almonds
¼ cup thinly sliced onion
¼ cup slivered green or red sweet pepper (or pimiento)
1 teaspoon tomato paste
¼ cup sherry or orange juice

Separate chicken pieces for frying, cutting off wing tips, neck, tail, giblets, and bony pieces of back. Use these to make broth: place in saucepan with ½ teaspoon of salt and 1½ cups of water; simmer for 30 minutes; strain and save broth for sauce.

Dust remaining chicken pieces with flour blended with salt, by shaking in a bag. Brown in butter, or mixture of butter and oil, and cook over moderately high heat, without crowding pan. Remove pieces and set aside as they are browned.

Add almonds to fat; stir-fry until nicely browned; remove and set aside. Add onion, cook until soft. Add green pepper, cook for 1 minute. Add tomato paste, sherry (or juice), and strained chicken broth. Replace chicken pieces and simmer uncovered for 20 minutes. Makes 4 servings.

Chicken and Dumplings

1 stewing chicken, cut up
Water
1 teaspoon salt, or to taste
1 medium onion, quartered, or 3 small white onions, peeled
1 cup whole-wheat flour

1½ teaspoons baking powder
¼ teaspoon salt
2 tablespoons soft shortening
1 egg, beaten
⅓ cup milk
Minced parsley

Place cut-up pieces of chicken in large heavy pot, such as a Dutch oven. Add water enough to almost but not quite cover chicken pieces. Add salt and onion. Cover, simmer until chicken is tender, 45 minutes–1 hour (an older chicken may require longer cooking). Or it can be cooked in a pressure cooker at 15 pounds for 15 minutes.

While chicken is cooking, prepare dumpling batter. Blend together flour, baking powder, and salt; cut in shortening. Add egg, then milk a little at a time, tossing with a fork, until mixture forms a sticky dough. When chicken is fork-tender, spoon dough over top of chicken pieces. Cover pot, bring liquid back to a boil (but do not put petcock on pressure cooker), and cook for 12 minutes. To serve, sprinkle chopped parsley over top. Spoon out onto plates, ladling broth over top of each serving of dumplings. Makes 6–8 servings.

Chicken Baked in Coconut Milk

Ordinarily, to make coconut milk shredded coconut is soaked in hot milk, then the milk is strained and the coconut thrown away. But in doing this, one is throwing away all the fiber, so I decided to experiment with keeping some of the coconut to see what might happen. I liked it. But the coconut swells up with soaking, and so much less coconut should be used. The other seasonings add zest to what could otherwise be a quite bland sauce.

1 3-pound chicken, cut up
½ teaspoon salt
½ teaspoon seasoned salt
Juice and grated rind of
  ½ lemon
½ teaspoon powdered cumin
2 garlic cloves, crushed
¼ teaspoon Tabasco sauce

1 cup milk, heated
¼ cup shredded dried
  coconut
2 tablespoons butter
1 cup water
1 tablespoon minced fresh
  dill, or 1 teaspoon dillweed

Cut chicken into 12 pieces, using poultry shears and a sharp knife. Remove as much skin and fat as possible. Put chicken pieces in shallow casserole; sprinkle all over (both sides) with salt and seasoned salt. Combine lemon juice and rind, cumin, crushed garlic, and Tabasco; pour over chicken pieces and marinate for 1 hour. Add hot milk to coconut, let stand. Dot chicken with butter, place in moderate oven (350° F.) for 20 minutes; turn each piece. To half the coconut-milk mixture add 1 cup of water and pour over chicken. Bake for 20 minutes longer, then add remaining coconut and milk. Bake for 10–15 minutes more, or until chicken pieces are nicely browned and coconut slightly browned. Just before serving, sprinkle dill over top of chicken. Makes 6 servings.

Chicken, Lima Bean, and Brown Rice Casserole

1 3-pound chicken, cut in 10 pieces
4 cups chicken broth
1 teaspoon bouquet garni (or any favorite herbs)
1 onion, quartered
3 tablespoons butter or margarine
½ teaspoon curry powder
Salt to taste
1½ cups brown rice (raw)
1 cup canned tomatoes, or 1 cup chopped fresh tomatoes
1 10-ounce package lima beans, thawed
12 pitted black olives

Separate tender pieces of chicken to use in casserole; make broth with wing tips, neck, etc., adding herbs and onion. Strain, measure, and set aside 4 cups. Brown chicken pieces in butter over high heat (in electric frying pan, set at 350°). As they cook, dust chicken pieces with salt and curry powder.

Add rice and stir to coat with fat. Add tomatoes; reduce heat (to 210° F. on electric frying pan). Add broth and limas. Cook, covered, until all liquid is absorbed (about 40–45 minutes). Before serving, place olives around top of rice. Makes 6 servings.

Note: Brown rice generally requires much longer cooking than long-grain white rice, but cooking time will vary. It may be cooked, and the water absorbed, within 35 minutes.

Poultry Stuffings

Apple Prune Poultry Stuffing

3 cups whole-wheat bread-crumbs
½ cup chopped dried prunes
2 apples (not peeled), chopped
½ cup chopped walnuts or toasted soybeans
¼ cup minced celery
2 slices bacon, cooked, crumbled, or 2 tablespoons vegetable protein bacon-bits
Salt, pepper
2 tablespoons sherry (optional)
2 tablespoons melted butter

Combine ingredients in order given. Makes enough for a 6-pound capon, a 5-pound duckling, or 2 broiler-size chickens. Double ingredients for a 10–12-pound turkey or goose.

Chestnut Stuffing

1½ pounds chestnuts in shell
6 celery stalks, diced
1 tablespoon celery leaves, minced
¼ cup shallots or scallion, chopped
4–5 tablespoons butter or margarine
1 teaspoon thyme or poultry seasoning

1 can water chestnuts, sliced and well drained
1 tablespoon salt
1 cup chopped apple, or ½ cup dried currants
6 cups stale whole-wheat or other whole-grain breadcrumbs
½ cup bran meal
¼ cup water (optional)

Slit shells of chestnuts by scoring with a small sharp knife; cook in boiling water for 30 minutes, or until slits in shell come open. Drain and cool. When they can be handled, remove the meat from shells, pare off brown skin, and chop.

Cook celery, celery leaves, and shallots or scallion in butter until soft. Add with seasonings, chestnuts, and fruit to breadcrumbs. Stir in bran meal. If a moist dressing is preferred, add water (though my family prefers the dressing to be moistened only with the turkey juices). Makes enough stuffing for a 10- or 12-pound turkey.

Spanish Stuffing for Turkey

½ pound lean pork, diced
3 tablespoons oil or drawn-out fat
1 medium onion, chopped
½ cup slivered almonds (or sunflower kernels)
½ pound fresh mushrooms, thoroughly washed and chopped
2 green peppers, seeded and chopped

½ cup raisins or currants
1 teaspoon thyme
½ teaspoon marjoram
½ cup minced parsley
Salt to taste
6 cups stale crumbs of oatmeal bread
2 eggs, beaten (optional)
¼ cup dry sherry (optional)

Brown pork in oil or fat, add onion and nuts, and stir-fry until lightly browned. Remove, put aside. Add remaining ingredients to pan, stir to blend with fat. Replace onions and nuts. Use as stuffing for a 12-pound turkey.

Fish and Other Seafood

Fish Poached in Coconut Milk

(LC)

Frozen fillets may be used for this dish—and with amazingly delicious results. Thaw fillets completely, cut into serving portions, and sprinkle with salt; let stand 15–20 minutes, then place in heavy saucepan or top-of-stove casserole. Sprinkle with freshly ground black pepper and a dash of cumin. Add milk barely to cover and about 2 tablespoons of shredded dried coconut. Cover pan or casserole, simmer over lowest possible heat about 15 minutes, or until fish flakes easily. Serve fish from pan or casserole onto plates; spoon coconut sauce over each serving, then sprinkle with chopped parsley.

Baked Sole au Gratin

(LC)

1-pound fillet of flounder or sole*	½ cup grated Parmesan cheese
½ cup milk	½ teaspoon salt
¼ cup finely crushed Shredded Wheat	¼ cup oil
	1 small onion, minced
2 tablespoons bran meal	1 lemon

Cut fish in serving portions (if frozen, sprinkle with salt and lemon juice and defrost completely at room temperature before baking). Soak fish in milk for 15 minutes; remove from milk, roll in mixture of crushed cereal, bran, cheese, and salt. Brush half the oil over bottom of shallow casserole, spread chopped onion over oil, then the fish over the onion. Sprinkle remaining cereal mixture over fish. Bake in moderately hot oven (375° F.) for 20 minutes, or until fish flakes easily. Serve with lemon wedges. Makes 3 or 4 servings.

*Cod or haddock may be used.

Baked Coconut Almond Cod
(LC)

Thaw a 1-pound package of frozen cod fillets. Sprinkle with salt and lemon juice, let stand for ½ hour before baking, then place in oiled shallow casserole over a layer of chopped onion. Sprinkle with oil (I use olive oil), top with ¼ cup each of chopped almonds and shredded coconut. Bake at 350° F. for 30 minutes, or until fish flakes easily. Makes 3 or 4 servings.

With nuts and apple: Instead of almonds and coconut, sprinkle top of fish with chopped dry-roasted peanuts and apple slices; dot with butter instead of sprinkling with oil.

Scalloped Oysters

1 pint (2 cups) shucked oysters
¼ cup oyster liquor
Lemon juice
½ cup (1 stick) margarine, melted
¼ cup rolled soy or triticale flakes
½ cup soft whole-wheat breadcrumbs
¾ teaspoon salt
¾ cup crushed Shredded Wheat or Triscuits
2 tablespoons cream

Drain oysters over a bowl to catch all the liquor. Sprinkle oysters with lemon juice. Melt margarine in frying pan, add flakes, and stir-fry until lightly browned; then add breadcrumbs and stir-fry till brown. Add ¾ teaspoon of salt and stir through the mixture. Turn off heat. Add crushed Shredded Wheat. (Taste for seasoning; it may need more salt.) Generously butter a 1-quart baking dish. First place a thin layer of the bread–cereal mixture over the bottom, then a layer of oysters, more cereal, etc., with the cereal mixture on top. Add cream to ¼ cup of oyster liquor; pour over top. Bake uncovered in oven preheated to 375° F. about 30 minutes, or until top is crisply browned. Makes 3 or 4 entree servings, or 6–8 side servings (with a turkey dinner). When served as an entree, nothing else is needed but a tossed salad and a light fruit dessert.

Shrimp Hawaiian

1½ cups shredded dried
   coconut
1 cup hot milk
2 tablespoons butter
½ cup minced scallion
1 small tomato, peeled,
   chopped
½ green pepper, diced

2 tablespoons soy flour
1 pound (16 ounces)
   frozen shelled shrimp,
   thawed
¼ cup macadamia nuts,
   chopped
Sliced papaya, avocado, or
   fresh pineapple

Soak 1 cup of the coconut in hot milk for ½ hour. Toast the remaining coconut to use as garnish. Squeeze out soaked coconut and reserve the coconut-flavored milk.

Melt butter, add scallion, tomato, and green pepper; cook about 2 minutes. Stir in flour, then add coconut milk. Cook until slightly thickened. Add thawed shrimp and nuts; transfer to a casserole. Bake, covered, in moderate (350° F.) oven for 30 minutes. Serve topped with toasted coconut, with fruit slices around the edges. Makes 6–8 servings.

Easy Crabmeat à la Russe

1 10-ounce can condensed
   cream of celery soup
½ cup sour cream
1 tablespoon horseradish
½ teaspoon dry mustard
¼ teaspoon celery seed
1 tablespoon sherry
1 cup cooked tiny peas
1 tablespoon chopped green
   pepper

1 cup crabmeat
4 slices lightly toasted oatmeal or whole-wheat bread
¼ cup coarsely crushed
   Wheat Chex blended with
   ½ tablespoon butter
2 tablespoons pine nuts or
   sunflower kernels

Blend together soup, sour cream, horseradish, and other seasonings, and sherry; heat, stirring, until heated through—do not boil. Add peas, green pepper, and crabmeat; continue to cook about 3 minutes longer. Serve hot over toasted bread with mixture of cereal and nuts over the top. Makes 4 servings.

CHAPTER 8

Exotic Dishes from Foreign Lands

The recipes collected in this chapter were chosen especially to show that food with good fiber content can also be enticing enough to serve to guests.

In Chinese and Japanese cuisine, vegetables are always cooked so briefly that they remain crisp, and only a small proportion of meat, poultry, or fish is needed. It is not necessary to prepare several different entrees to serve a Chinese meal—why not adapt Chinese cooking to the American pattern and serve just one entree, accompanied by rice (or millet).

The cuisines of many foreign countries give a prominent place to legumes, and from them we can learn new and intriguing ways to prepare these high-fiber high-protein members of the plant family. Nuts, another good source of fiber and protein, are also frequently included as ingredients in foreign cookery.

A number of rice casseroles are included; those who prefer to use brown rice may do so, but will need to allow a longer cooking time. However, as was pointed out previously, converted white rice has almost exactly the same protein and mineral content as brown rice, and neither brown rice nor other rice products (except pure rice bran) have significant fiber content.

For those seeking more fiber, millet grains may be substituted for rice. This will work in almost every one of the rice recipes that follow. Use the same measure of millet but more liquid: for each cup of millet grains (*not* millet meal), you will need 3 cups of water as opposed to the 2 cups of water per cup of rice.

In some cases, I have departed from the original recipes and have "snuck in" some extra fiber in one form or another.

Cantonese Pork with Cauliflower
(LC)

½ pound lean pork, cut in ½-inch cubes
Lemon juice
5 tablespoons oil (approx.)
1 large garlic clove, cut in quarters
2 cups small flowerlets of cauliflower
1 cup sliced fresh mushrooms
Inner stem and leaves of cauliflower, cut in 2-inch pieces, or 2 stalks bok choy
½ cup green pepper, in chunks
¼ cup chopped fresh coriander or fresh fennel, chopped
3 thin slices ginger root, minced, or ½ teaspoon ground ginger
2 scallions, white and part of the green, sliced
Salt
1 tablespoon soy sauce
1 tablespoon sherry
1 tablespoon whole-bran cereal
½ cup water
½ cup peanuts or toasted soybeans

Sprinkle pork with lemon juice. Heat 3 tablespoons of oil in wok or heavy frying pan. Add garlic clove, cook until golden and soft (about 30 seconds); crush with fork to release juice into oil, then remove. Add cauliflower to oil, stir-fry about 2 minutes. Add mushrooms, cook for 1 minute. Add cauliflower leaves, green pepper, coriander (or fennel), ginger, and scallions; stir-fry 1 or 2 minutes longer. Sprinkle with salt from shaker as vegetables cook. Remove vegetables with slotted spoon.

Add more oil to pan and sauté pieces of pork until golden, stirring occasionally. Blend together soy sauce, sherry, and bran; let stand while pork is cooking. Replace vegetables in pan, thin bran mixture with water and add to pan; add nuts or soybeans. Cook until ingredients are heated through and sauce is slightly thickened. Serve with hot cooked millet. Makes 4 servings.

Note: A topping of shredded coconut may be added just before serving, if desired.

Shrimp with Cauliflower

(LC)

Instead of pork in the previous recipe, use 6 ounces shelled shrimp. Green peas and celery cabbage may be used instead of cauliflower and the cauliflower leaves, if preferred.

Moo Goo Gai Pan

(LC)

2 whole chicken breasts
Salt, pepper
3 tablespoons oil
½ cup blanched whole almonds
3 scallions, minced
1 cup thinly sliced mushrooms
1 cup diced seeded green pepper

3 or 4 thin slices green ginger root, or ¼ teaspoon ground ginger
1 cup frozen tiny peas, thawed
2 teaspoons cornstarch or arrowroot
¼ cup chicken broth or water
2 tablespoons dry sherry
2 tablespoons soy sauce

Skin and bone chicken breasts, cut into 1-inch pieces. Sprinkle chicken with salt and pepper. Heat oil, quickly sauté chicken until meat turns solidly white (about 3 or 4 minutes). Remove from pan. Add whole blanched almonds and stir-fry until nicely browned. Remove. Add scallions, mushrooms, green pepper, and ginger; stir-fry for 2 minutes. Add peas, stir until broken up and coated with oil; cook for 2 minutes. Dissolve cornstarch in some of chicken broth, add remaining broth, sherry, and soy sauce. Replace chicken and almonds in pan; cook, stirring, until sauce is thickened and smooth (about 4 minutes longer). Serve by itself as an entree or as part of a multi-dish Chinese dinner. As a single entree, it will serve 3 or 4 persons; as part of a multi-entree dinner, 6–8.

Stir-Fried Shrimp with Broccoli

(LC)

6 ounces medium-to-large frozen shelled shrimp, defrosted
1 tablespoon whole-wheat flour or arrowroot
1 egg white, unbeaten
½ teaspoon salt
1 tablespoon water
4 tablespoons oil

1 10-ounce package baby broccoli spears, thawed, or fresh broccoli cut in small pieces
3 stalks bok choy or celery, cut in 1-inch pieces
2 scallions, chopped
½ cup almonds, peanuts, or cashew nuts
Salt to taste

The shrimp should be patted dry with paper towel, as should the frozen thawed broccoli—otherwise they will not cook as quickly in the oil. Dip shrimp in mixture of flour (or arrowroot), egg white, salt, and water. Let stand for 5 minutes.

Heat oil in wok or deep heavy skillet. Add broccoli spears, stir-fry about 2 minutes. Add bok choy or celery and scallions; cook for 1 minute. Sprinkle with salt as they cook. Remove with slotted spoon.

Add the batter-dipped shrimp to the hot oil; cook until golden-brown on all sides, turning once or twice. Replace vegetables, add nuts. Cook about 2 minutes longer. Serve sprinkled with nuts. Makes 4–6 servings.

Note: Soy sauce is not added during cooking and should not be needed. However, it can be passed at the table for those who want it.

Arabian Baked Chicken

(LC)

12 chicken legs, disjointed
2 teaspoons seasoned salt
1 teaspoon garlic salt
1 teaspoon ground nutmeg
½ teaspoon cinnamon or crushed cardamom
1 teaspoon thyme leaves
¼ cup olive oil

2 large Spanish onions, sliced
½ cup chopped dried apricots or dried currants
¼ cup chopped dates
8 carrots, scraped, cut in strips
½ cup chopped peanuts

Season the chicken pieces with the two kinds of salt, the spices and thyme. Sauté in olive oil until nicely browned on all sides. Place chicken in large casserole in layers with onion and fruit. Cover and bake in a moderate (350° F.) oven for 45 minutes. Cook carrots briefly (about 2 minutes). Drain, add with nuts to casserole, cover once more and bake another 20 minutes, or until chicken is fork-tender. Serves 12.

Roast Chicken Karachi

(LC)

1 5-pound roasting chicken or 6- to 7-pound capon
1 lemon
Salt
3 cups partially cooked bulgur
1 cup frozen tiny peas (not cooked)
2 tablespoons blanched toasted almonds or sunflower kernels

¼ cup raisins or chopped dried apricots
1 cup plain yogurt
2 tablespoons minced ginger root, or 1 teaspoon powdered ginger
2 tablespoons grated onion

Prepare chicken for roasting by rinsing out cavity; sprinkle inside and out with salt from shaker. Rub skin with cut side of lemon, then squeeze lemon for juice and sprinkle juice in cavity. Make broth with chicken trimmings and giblets to use for gravy.

For the stuffing, combine bulgur (cooked only about 12 minutes), uncooked frozen peas, nuts and fruit. Add salt and other seasonings to taste. Stuff chicken cavity *loosely:* it will swell as bulgur continues to cook. Truss.

Rub or brush outside of chicken with mixture of yogurt, ginger, and grated onion. Bake in shallow roasting pan in moderate oven (350° F.) about 1 hour, or until leg moves easily. Yogurt gives chicken very golden crisp exterior. Serves 6–8.

Indonesian Pork and Chicken

(LC)

1 pound lean raw pork, cut in slivers
2 tablespoons oil
3 whole chicken breasts, cut in 2-inch pieces
1 cup chopped onion
1½ cups celery or bok choy, sliced diagonally
1 tablespoon curry powder
⅛ teaspoon ground ginger
⅛ teaspoon cayenne

1 cup fresh bean sprouts
3 water chestnuts, sliced
1 cup snow peas or thinly sliced broccoli
1 tablespoon cornstarch or arrowroot
3 tablespoons soy sauce
½ cup chicken broth
1 cup coconut milk
1 cup chopped peanuts
Hot cooked rice or millet

Sauté pork in hot oil until well browned; remove. Add chicken, cook until nicely browned on all sides; remove. Add onion and celery or bok choy; stir-fry about 3 minutes. Add seasonings; stir to blend. Add bean sprouts, water chestnuts, and snow peas (or broccoli). Stir-fry until barely tender—still crisp (about 3 or 4 minutes). Replace pork and chicken. Blend cornstarch with soy sauce and broth; stir into wok or pan, bring to a boil, and cook until almost dry. Add strained coconut milk. Simmer, stirring, until sauce is smooth and thickened. Add peanuts, or serve peanuts over top as garnish. Serve accompanied by rice or millet. Makes about 6 servings.

Szechuan-Style Chicken

(LC)

2 whole chicken breasts, skinned, boned, and diced
¼ cup oil (approx.)
2 teaspoons arrowroot or cornstarch
2 tablespoons water
1 egg white, unbeaten
4 scallions, sliced
3 stalks bok choy, chopped, or 1 cup coarsely chopped celery cabbage

1 green pepper, cut in large pieces
3 paper-thin slices ginger root
5 tablespoons soy sauce
2 tablespoons dry sherry
1 teaspoon salt
¼ teaspoon cayenne
1 cup dry-roasted peanuts

Chicken should be cut into bite-size pieces, then tossed with a mixture of cornstarch blended with water and egg white. Set aside.

Heat 2 tablespoons of oil in wok or deep frying pan. Add scallions, bok choy, and green pepper. Cook for 2 minutes; remove and keep warm.

Fry chicken pieces in oil, adding more oil if necessary. Stir-fry until it is crisply browned. Mince ginger root. Add to mixture of soy sauce, sherry, salt, and cayenne. (The cayenne is essential—this dish is supposed to be quite spicy.) Replace vegetables in pan, add peanuts, then add soy-sherry mixture, and stir and cook about 1 minute longer. Makes 4–6 servings.

Beef Chimechanges

Wheat or Corn Tortillas
¾ pound lean ground beef
1 large onion, chopped
Oil
1 green pepper, seeded and chopped
1 teaspoon crushed dried red-hot chili peppers
1 garlic clove, minced
½ teaspoon salt
½ teaspoon cumin

1 tablespoon chopped fresh coriander, or 1 teaspoon dried cilantro or chopped parsley
½ cup cooked or refried black beans
Guacamole
Green Chili Relish
Shredded lettuce
Goat cheese or feta cheese

Prepare tortillas (see recipe on page 57). To prepare the fillings, sauté the beef and onion in 2 tablespoons of oil until meat loses its pink color. And green pepper, chili peppers, garlic, seasonings and herbs. Stir-fry about 5 minutes longer. Spoon ¼ cup of meat mixture into each tortilla, fold over ends, then the sides, to form an enclosed packet; fasten with picks. (If tortillas have been made ahead and are too brittle to fold over easily, sprinkle lightly with water, wrap with foil, and heat in oven about 15 minutes.) Fry three or four of these packets at a time in hot oil to brown on each side. Drain on absorbent paper, keep warm in warming oven (200° F.) until time to serve. Serve over shredded lettuce with Guacamole (page 72), Green Chili Relish, refried beans, and cheese as accompaniments. Makes about 18.

Note: Instead of tortillas, the mixture can be enclosed in very thin crepes made with whole-wheat pancake mix, using 1 cup of liquid to ½ cup of mix: use a 7-inch skillet or crepe pan and tilt so batter spreads out to edges. Turn as soon as firm. Brush tops with oil, bake in 400° F. oven until browned.

Green Chili Relish

3 medium slightly green tomatoes, chopped
3 green chilis, seeded and diced
½ cup chopped onion
½ cup chopped sweet green pepper
1 teaspoon vinegar
Salt, pepper
Dash of cayenne or Tabasco

Combine all ingredients; marinate at least 1 hour before serving. Makes about 1½ cups.

Mexican Chicken with Fruit

(LC)

1 3-pound fryer, cut up
¼–½ cup whole-wheat flour
1 teaspoon salt
3 or 4 tablespoons shortening or oil
1 cup minced fresh onion
2 garlic cloves, minced
¼ teaspoon dried hot chili pepper
½ green pepper, seeded and diced
1 cup diced fresh pineapple, or 1 small can unsweetened pineapple chunks, drained
2 cups chicken broth
⅓ cup raisins
Hot cooked rice
¼ cup blanched toasted almonds
1 cup sliced papaya
1 avocado, peeled and sliced

Separate trimmings and giblets of chicken from the rest; use to make broth. Dust remaining chicken pieces with mixture of flour and salt. Brown in 3 tablespoons of shortening or oil. Remove to a large shallow casserole. To same pan add onion, garlic, and chili pepper with remaining oil, if needed. Cook until soft. Add green pepper and pineapple, cook for 1 minute. Sprinkle 2 tablespoons of the flour-salt mixture over the vegetables, stir to blend well. Add chicken broth (made with trimmings) and raisins; simmer until broth is somewhat thickened. Pour over chicken in casserole. Bake uncovered in moderate (350° F.) oven about 1 hour, or until chicken is very tender. Serve on a large platter over a mound of cooked rice, topped with a sprinkling of toasted almonds, and with slices of papaya and avocado around the edge. Makes 6 servings.

Note: Instead of papaya, orange segments or thin slices of cantaloupe may be used with the avocado.

Kibbe
(Middle Eastern Meatloaf)   (LC)

1½ cups fine bulgur	2 teaspoons salt
2 or 3 large onions	¼–½ teaspoon freshly ground
2 pounds lean lamb, ground	pepper
fine	¼ cup olive oil or melted
	butter

Place bulgur in bowl; cover with cold water. With hands, lift from water and press out liquid, then knead into compact shape.

Put onions through medium blade of food grinder or beat in blender until nearly pureed. Put meat on wooden board, pound with mallet or rolling pin to make it paste-like. Pound onion, salt, and pepper into meat, then add bulgur. Beat and knead until mixture is very smooth. (Moisten palms of hands with water so meat will not stick.) Divide into two parts. Press half in the bottom of an oiled 9x17x2-inch baking pan. Cover with the following stuffing:

½ cup pine nuts or sunflower	½ teaspoon salt
kernels	¼ teaspoon pepper
½ pound lean lamb, ground	¼ cup olive oil or melted
	butter

Cover with remaining bulgur mixture, pressing into an even layer. Score top into diamond-shape pattern with small sharp knife; brush olive oil or melted butter over top. Bake in oven preheated to 400° F. (hot) until top is crisply browned (about 40 minutes). Makes 8 servings.

Kibbe Meatballs

Prepare the same bulgur mixture as in preceding recipe, but form into large balls, about 2 inches in diameter, and press pine nuts into center of each, then close over opening. Brown in hot olive oil or butter on all sides, or brush with oil or butter and bake in hot oven until browned. Serve with mint-flavored plain yogurt as a sauce.

Rice Limeno

This is a very unusual rice casserole from Peru or Colombia (I'm not sure which).

¼ cup blanched slivered almonds
4 tablespoons oil
1 small onion, chopped
1 garlic clove, minced
1 green pepper, seeded and minced
½ teaspoon dried crushed hot chili pepper
1 3-ounce jar diced pimiento, drained
1¼ cups converted long-grain rice
2½ cups water
1 teaspoon salt
1 cup shelled or frozen peas, or baby limas

2 tablespoons chopped prunes or dried currants
12 slices veal scallopini, or 1 pound lean pork cut in small cubes
1 tablespoon whole-wheat flour blended with ½ teaspoon salt
3 tablespoons butter
½ cup sherry (or ¼ cup orange juice, ¼ cup water)
½ cup beef bouillon
Minced parsley
Pimiento-stuffed green olives

Sauté nuts in oil until lightly browned; remove, set aside. Add to oil the onion, garlic, green pepper, chili pepper, and pimiento; stir-fry until onion is golden. Add rice, stir to coat with oil. Add water, salt, peas or limas, and prunes or currants. Cover, bring to a boil, reduce heat; cook over lowest heat until water is absorbed (about 20 minutes). Spoon into large (3-quart) casserole.

Pound veal slices with edge of small plate, working in flour and salt; if pork is used, shake pieces in bag with flour mixture. Sauté meat quickly in butter until browned. Add sherry (or orange juice and water), simmer for 1 or 2 minutes, and remove meat. Cook until liquid is reduced by half, then add broth, and simmer, stirring, until all bits have been loosened from bottom of pan. Place meat around edges of casserole over rice mixture; cover both meat and rice with sauce. Place nuts and parsley over center, the olives around the meat. Keep warm in oven, covered, until time to serve. Serves 6 generously.

Lebanese Pilaf

1 pound boned lamb, cut in small pieces	¼ teaspoon cinnamon
	¼ teaspoon black pepper
2 tablespoons butter or olive oil	½ cup chopped dried apricots
2 large onions, chopped	½ cup currants or raisins
1 cup converted long-grain rice	¼ cup shelled pistachio nuts or pine nuts
2 cups cooked or canned chickpeas, well drained	2 cups beef broth or water
1½ teaspoons salt	1½ tablespoons melted butter
½ teaspoon thyme	3 tablespoons lemon juice
	Chopped parsley

Sauté meat slowly in butter until well browned (about 20 minutes). Remove. Add onions to fat in pan, cook until soft. Add rice, stir to coat with oil. Add seasonings, chickpeas, fruit, and nuts; add broth, bring to a boil, then lower heat and cook, covered, for 20 minutes, or until all liquid is absorbed. Combine melted butter and lemon juice, sprinkle over top of rice; top with parsley. A marvelous and inexpensive company dish. Serves 6.

Bulgur Pilaf

Instead of rice, use 1 cup of bulgur in above recipe, add 1 cup of canned tomatoes.

Greek Lamb Stew with Okra
(LC)

3 pounds lamb for stew
   (with bone)
2–3 tablespoons olive oil
1 medium onion, sliced
1½ cups tomato juice
¼ teaspoon thyme

1 teaspoon salt
1 pound fresh okra, or 1
   10-ounce package frozen
   okra
1 teaspoon lemon juice

Lamb for stew is usually precut and prepackaged, or you may request the butcher to cut lamb shanks or shoulder for you.

Brown meat in oil; push to one side, lower heat, add onion to pan, and cook until soft. Add tomato juice, thyme, and salt. Bring to a boil, lower heat, cook covered until meat is very tender (about 1½ hours). Skim fat from top of broth. During last 5 minutes, add okra; it should still be just a little crisp when served. Sprinkle lemon juice over stew just before serving. A lovely combination of flavors. Serves 4.

Cochifrito

2 pounds boneless lamb, or
   3½ pounds lamb with
   bone, cut for stew
¼ cup whole-wheat or soy
   flour
2 teaspoons salt
3–4 tablespoons olive oil
1 garlic clove, slit
1 tablespoon minced parsley
1 teaspoon paprika

1 cup water
½ teaspoon dried mint,
   crushed
Grated rind and juice of ½
   lemon
10–12 baby artichokes,
   trimmed, quartered, or 1
   package frozen artichoke
   hearts

Lamb should be cut into cubes, if boneless; with bone, cut into serving portions. Dredge meat with flour mixed with salt. Brown in hot oil; remove from pan as pieces are browned. Place garlic in oil, cook until golden and soft; press with tines of fork to release garlic juice into oil, then remove shreds of garlic. Add parsley and paprika to pan, stir to blend. Add water, mint, and lemon juice and rind. Cover and simmer until meat is tender (1½ to 2 hours). Add baby artichokes during last half hour, the frozen artichokes during last 10 minutes. Continue to cook until artichokes are tender. Makes 5 or 6 servings.

Pork and Beans Guimaraes
(A specialty of northern Portugal)

1 pound honeycomb tripe, ready to cook	3 or 4 onions, peeled and quartered
1 pound dried marrow or navy beans, presoaked	½ cup chopped ham
	8–10 cups water
½ pound boned pork, cubed	2–3 teaspoons salt
2 or 3 carrots, scraped and cubed	1 tablespoon paprika
	1–1½ teaspoons cumin

Tripe of any kind is not easy to find in American markets and if it cannot be found, use chicken legs instead. When available, honeycomb tripe is the most desirable, especially if it has been tenderized; otherwise, it may require 10 or 12 hours of cooking.

Drain soaked beans; place in large kettle (or crock-pot) with tripe (or chicken legs) and remaining ingredients. Cook covered over very low heat for 3–4 hours. It may be necessary to add more water from time to time. Or it can be cooked in a bean-pot in the oven overnight, at 275° F. The cumin is what gives the stew its unique flavor. Makes 8–10 servings.

Pork and Celery Root Avgolemono

2–3 pounds lean pork, cubed	1½ cups water or chicken broth
6 tablespoons butter or margarine	1 tablespoon minced parsley
2 medium onions, sliced	1 large celery root (celeriac)
2 tablespoons whole-wheat or soy flour	4 egg yolks
1½ teaspoons salt, or to taste	4 tablespoons lemon juice

Brown pork in butter; push to one side of pan or remove meat. Add onions, cook until soft and golden without browning. Stir in flour and salt, cook until flour mixture bubbles. Slowly stir in water or chicken broth (if using broth, use less salt). Simmer covered for 1 hour. Meantime, peel celeriac and cut into slivers. Place over meat in casserole; continue to cook ½ hour longer, or until both meat and celeriac are very tender.

Beat egg yolks until thick and lighter in color; with whisk, beat in lemon juice 1 tablespoon at a time. Add a few tablespoons of the hot broth to the mixture; beat until smooth. Then stir egg mixture into sauce in the casserole. Turn off heat; keep covered on stove until time to serve. (If dinner is delayed, keep covered in warming oven.) Makes 6–8 servings.

Note: If celeriac is not available locally, Pascal celery can be used: you will need at least 3 cups of celery, sliced in 2-inch pieces at an angle.

Crepes Florentine

CREPE BATTER:
- ¾ cup buttermilk pancake mix
- ¼ cup bran meal
- 2 eggs, beaten
- 1½ cups milk
- 1 teaspoon oil or melted butter

FILLING AND SAUCE:
- 1½ cups chopped spinach
- 2 tablespoons butter
- 2 tablespoons soy flour
- 1 cup milk
- Salt to taste
- 1 egg yolk
- ½ cup shredded Swiss cheese
- 2 tablespoons chopped sunflower kernels
- ⅓ cup slivered toasted almonds

Prepare crepe batter beforehand: combine ingredients in a bowl, beat just until well blended and the consistency of cream. Refrigerate for 1–2 hours.

Meantime, prepare filling. Either fresh or frozen chopped spinach may be used, but if using fresh spinach, cook just until limp (about 1 minute). Do not cook the frozen spinach at all. Press out every bit of liquid: *this is important.* To make sauce, melt butter, stir in flour, cook until it bubbles, then slowly add milk and salt to taste. Remove from heat, beat in egg yolk. Add half the sauce and half the cheese to the spinach; stir in the sunflower kernels. Use mixture as filling.

Cook crepes in a 7-inch skillet: melt enough butter to cover bottom of pan; pour in 2 tablespoons of batter, tilt so batter covers pan. As soon as lightly browned on bottom, flip, cook on the other side. Repeat, making 12 crepes. Put 2 tablespoons of filling in each, roll up, place stuffed crepes in greased shallow baking dish with overlapped side down. Cover with remaining sauce; top with almonds. Bake at 375° F. until almonds are toasted and sauce lightly browned and bubbly. Makes 12 crepes; serves 4.

Boerijch

1 pound dried black-eyed peas, or 3 boxes frozen black-eyed peas
Salted water
2 medium onions, chopped
¼ cup olive oil
1 teaspoon salt
1 teaspoon orange blossom honey
½ cup tomato sauce
1 cup chopped nuts
½ cup water
¼ cup minced parsley

Cook dried peas (without presoaking) very slowly in salted water until tender, adding more water as necessary as they cook. (This may take 3 or 4 hours.) Drain peas when quite tender. (Or cook frozen peas according to package directions; drain.)

Cook onion in olive oil until soft; add salt, honey, tomato sauce, nuts, the cooked peas, water, and parsley. Simmer for 10–15 minutes. Good either hot or cold (but not chilled). Makes 8–10 servings.

Kichri

9 peppercorns
¼ teaspoon crushed cardamom
⅛ teaspoon ground cloves
¼ teaspoon allspice
1 tablespoon butter or oil
½ cup chopped onion
⅓ cup brown rice
1 tablespoon lemon juice
1 teaspoon salt
3 cups water
⅓ cup brown lentils

Crush spices together with mortar and pestle or in blender. Add to butter in a large heavy pot. Stir in onion and cook slowly until onions are soft and golden (about 3 minutes). Add rice, stir to blend with butter, then add lemon juice, salt, and water. Bring to a boil and cook covered for 10 minutes. Add lentils and continue to cook over lowest heat until lentils are tender but not soft. Makes 2 cups or 4 servings.

Falafel

1 cup dried chickpeas (garbanzos)	1½ teaspoons salt
¼ cup parsley or fresh coriander	½ teaspoon cumin
½ cup chopped onion	¼ teaspoon freshly ground black pepper
1 garlic clove, minced	2 tablespoons water
¼ cup lemon juice	Oil for frying

Soak chickpeas in water to cover *for 24 hours*. Drain; put through food grinder with parsley, onion, and garlic. Mix with lemon juice, salt, cumin, pepper, and water. Form mixture into balls by scooping with a tablespoon.

Heat oil, 2 inches deep, until it will brown a cube of bread in 30 seconds. Drop chickpea mixture carefully into the oil to avoid spattering and do not crowd pan. Fry until brown on all sides, turning once. Lift out with slotted spoon. Serve hot as an appetizer or as part of a vegetarian dinner. Makes 18–20.

(Falafel is a Middle Eastern specialty, popular in Egypt, Israel, Lebanon, and all the other countries round about. The hot croquettes are often served with yogurt.)

Musur-Gos is a specialty at the Velha Goa Restaurant in Lisbon. Like most Indian food, it is quite spicy, but the coriander gives it an aromatic quality that is delightful.

Musur-Gos
(Goa-Style Lentils with Meat)

CURRY MIXTURE:

¼ cup chopped fresh coriander
2 garlic cloves
Several thin slices green ginger, minced
1 teaspoon cumin

¾ teaspoon black peppercorns, crushed
3 green peppers, seeded and chopped
1 teaspoon dried chili peppers, crushed
¼ teaspoon nutmeg

Put all the above ingredients in a blender and beat until smooth. Set aside.

2 pounds boned meat (veal or beef), cut in small cubes
2 teaspoons salt
¼ teaspoon pepper
1 garlic clove, crushed
2 tablespoons vinegar
4 large onions, sliced
3 or 4 tablespoons oil

2 tablespoons chopped coriander
1 pound lentils, cooked separately
6 medium tomatoes, seeded and chopped
Vinegar and salt to taste

Place cut-up meat in bowl; add mixture of salt, pepper, garlic, and vinegar; toss to blend. Marinate at least ½ hour. Cook onions slowly in oil until soft and golden; add meat, brown lightly. Add the curry mixture and more chopped coriander. Then add cooked lentils and just enough water to barely cover mixture; finally add tomatoes. Cook slowly, uncovered, until meat is very tender. Add a dash or two of vinegar at the end and taste for salt. Serve with rice or cooked millet. Makes 8–10 servings.

CHAPTER 9

Economy Casseroles and Vegetarian Entrees

There's increasing evidence that an excess of meat in the diet can be injurious to health. It may contribute to high blood pressure, strokes, heart attack, certain types of cancer, and atherosclerosis. The minimum daily allowance of protein required by most adults is only 14 grams—and one can get this much from a single plump hamburger or 1½ ounces of tuna.

When the source of protein is primarily meat, it is possible to have too much. A report of the American Cancer Society (May, 1975) concludes that rich meats and animal fats appear to overstimulate the body's hormonal system, which is regarded as a factor in breast and uterine cancer.

Today vegetarianism is enjoying unprecedented popularity in this country, and innovative vegetarians are doing the rest of us a favor in demonstrating how interesting meatless meals can be. But even if you don't go all the way to vegetarianism, serving vegetable entrees frequently and cutting down the proportion of meat in casseroles have a further advantage: an appreciable saving on the grocery bill!

Since turkey is one of the most economical of meat buys, there are various recipes in this chapter using leftover turkey to provide many imaginative meals.

Cocido con Pavo

Leftover roast turkey
1½ quarts water
Salt
2 or 3 onions, quartered
1 celery stalk, with leaves
1 cup leftover turkey dressing (if made with whole-
  grain bread)
1 pound (2 cups) dried
  chickpeas (garbanzos),
  soaked
½ cup chopped onion

3 garlic cloves, minced
2 tablespoons olive oil
1 can (1 pound) tomatoes
½ cup chopped cooked ham
¼ cup chopped Italian
  parsley
1 pound sweet potatoes,
  peeled and cubed
1 cup finely chopped
  collard greens
Hard-cooked eggs for
garnish

Trim carcass of turkey and set aside all meat. Place carcass in kettle (broken in pieces), add water, 1 tablespoon of salt, onion, and celery. Cover; simmer for 1 hour. Strain; measure 6 cups.

Return strained broth to kettle with leftover dressing and drained soaked chickpeas. Cook onion and garlic in oil until soft; add tomatoes and cook for 5 minutes. Transfer mixture to kettle with turkey broth. Bring to a boil, cook covered 2½–3 hours, or until garbanzos are tender. Add ham, reserved turkey meat, parsley, sweet potatoes, and collard greens. Continue to cook about ½ hour longer. Serve garnished with chopped hard-cooked egg and additional minced parsley. Makes 8–10 servings.

Baked Turkey Hash

3 cups chopped cooked
  turkey
2 cups crumbled Shredded
  Wheat
¼ cup sunflower kernels
1 cup turkey gravy or canned
  chicken gravy
½ cup chopped celery
1 tablespoon minced parsley

2 eggs, slightly beaten
1 tablespoon lemon juice
1 teaspoon grated lemon rind
3 tablespoons minced onion,
  or 1 teaspoon instant
  minced onion
1 pimiento, chopped
¾ cup milk
Salt, pepper to taste

Combine all ingredients in large bowl, turn into lightly greased shallow baking dish, about 12x7 inches. Place this in a larger roasting pan to which water is added to depth of ¼ inch. Bake in moderate oven (350° F.) for 50–60 minutes. Cut in squares to serve. Good with creamed cauliflower and frenched green beans. Makes 8–10 servings.

(For 3 or 4 servings, divide all ingredients by approximately ⅓ and use 1 egg. Exact measurements are not necessary.)

Chicken (or Turkey) Pie

8 very small white onions, cooked or canned
2 cups cut-up chicken or turkey
1 package (10-ounce) frozen peas and carrots
1 3-ounce can mushroom crowns, or 6–8 button mushrooms, trimmed
1 can condensed cream of chicken soup
Milk
3 tablespoons bran meal or whole-bran cereal
Biscuit or pastry dough for 1 crust

If using fresh or frozen whole onions, parboil first, saving the cooking liquid. Combine cooked or canned drained onions with chicken, peas and carrots (need not be precooked), and drained mushrooms. Place mixture in 8-inch-square baking dish. For sauce, combine soup, reserved onion liquid, and liquid from canned mushrooms plus milk, if needed, for desired consistency (it should be fairly thin). Stir in bran; pour over chicken (or turkey) mixture. For the crust, use Oat Biscuit Dough, Hi-Fiber Pastry for 1 crust, or 1 stick of pie crust mix (working in a little bran). Makes 1 pie, 4 servings.

Turkey Pom-Poms

2 cups cooked millet or pink lentils
½ cup diced celery
½ cup chopped walnuts or sunflower "nuts"
2 tablespoons minced onion
¾ teaspoon salt
¾ teaspoon thyme or poultry seasoning
2 cups cooked diced turkey
¼ cup melted butter
2 eggs, slightly beaten
¾ cup fine dry whole-wheat crumbs, or finely crushed whole-wheat or bran breakfast cereal
Mushroom Sauce

When cooking millet or pink lentils, add extra water and cook until very soft, with all liquid absorbed. Combine with celery, nuts, onion, seasonings, and turkey. Stir in butter and eggs. Shape into 2-inch balls and roll in crumbs or crushed cereal. Arrange in a lightly greased baking pan or baking sheet. Bake in preheated oven (425° F.) for 30 minutes, or until crisp and brown on the outside. Makes 6–8 servings.

Mushroom Sauce

Sauté 1 cup of sliced fresh mushrooms in 2 tablespoons of butter or margarine until nicely browned. Stir in 2 tablespoons of whole-wheat or soy flour, cook for 2 minutes; slowly stir in 2 cups of chicken broth (made with concentrate). Simmer for 10 minutes until smooth and thickened. Remove from heat; stir in ¼ cup of plain yogurt.

The combination of rice and chickpeas appears in the cuisines of many Mediterranean countries. The following is a specialty in the Spanish city of Valencia.

Rosetxat

¼ cup olive oil
1 garlic clove
2 fully ripe tomatoes, chopped, or 2 canned peeled tomatoes, drained (save juice for broth)
1 medium onion, chopped
2 tablespoons minced parsley
¼ cup lean ham, minced
1 teaspoon paprika

½ pound butifarra or Italian sweet sausage, cut in 1-inch lengths
1 teaspoon salt
2 cups canned or cooked chickpeas, drained
1 cup long-grain converted rice
¼ teaspoon saffron, in 1 cup boiling beef broth

Heat olive oil, add garlic, and cook until soft; then mash garlic into oil with tines of fork. Add tomato, onion, parsley, ham, and paprika. Cook until onion is soft and ham lightly browned. Add sausage and brown lightly. Add salt, chickpeas, and rice. To boiling-hot saffron-flavored broth, add juice from tomatoes, liquid from canned garbanzos, or water to make a total of 2 cups of liquid. Add this to rice mixture. Transfer to deep casserole; complete cooking, covered, in moderate oven until all liquid is absorbed (about 30 minutes longer). Makes 6 servings.

Stuffed Zucchini

(LC)

4 zucchini, each 6–8 inches long
¾ pound lean ground beef
¼ cup finely crushed whole-bran cereal
1 or 2 garlic cloves, crushed
2 tablespoons minced parsley
1 teaspoon salt
¼ cup olive oil

3 slices stale whole-wheat or health bread
1 cup water
1 teaspoon paprika
5 or 6 toasted sunflower kernels, minced
1 hard-cooked egg, yolk and white separated
1 tablespoon tomato paste

Scrape the squash very lightly with edge of a sharp paring knife, cut lengthwise slice from each, then scoop out the centers, making each into a boat shape. Blend removed zucchini pulp with meat, bran, garlic, 1 tablespoon of parsley, and salt. Stuff into squash "boats." Form meatballs of remaining meat mixture.

In a skillet, brown both the meatballs and the outside of the stuffed squash in olive oil, quickly, without cooking through. Transfer to a top-of-stove casserole or large saucepan. In same skillet, fry the stale bread in olive oil until crisp on both sides; remove from oil, place in bowl containing 1 cup of water. Pour off all but 2 tablespoons of olive oil from skillet; add to skillet paprika, sunflower kernels, egg yolk (which has been forced through a fine sieve), and tomato paste, then add the bread with the water in which it soaked. Simmer this mixture for 5 minutes to form a sauce. Pour sauce over squash and meatballs in casserole; cover. Simmer over low heat or bake in oven preheated to 350° F. for 20–30 minutes longer. Sprinkle with remaining minced parsley and minced egg white. Serve with baked potatoes and a salad. Makes 4 servings.

Tuna Noodle Casserole

4 cups cooked whole-wheat noodles
1 can (6 or 7 ounces) chunk-style tuna, drained
3 hard-cooked eggs, chopped
¼ cup sunflower kernels or toasted soybeans
1 10-ounce package frozen limas, thawed, not cooked
1 10½-ounce can condensed tomato soup
1 10½-ounce can condensed beef bouillon
1 teaspoon horseradish
8 pitted black olives, sliced
½ cup crushed Shredded Wheat
½ cup shredded Swiss or American cheese

Cook whole-wheat noodles in rapidly boiling salted water until tender; drain (2 cups before cooking makes 4 cups cooked). Divide in thirds; arrange ⅓ in bottom of greased 1½-quart casserole.

Combine all remaining ingredients but Shredded Wheat and cheese. Place half of mixture over noodles, add more noodles, remaining tuna mixture, and remaining noodles. Combine crushed cereal and cheese; spread over top. Bake at 375° F. for 30–40 minutes until cheese is melted and sauce bubbling. Makes 4–6 servings.

Pastel de Choclo
(Chilean Corn Pie)

½ cup diced cooked chicken
2 cups lean boneless pork, cooked and diced
1½ cups white sweet corn, scraped from cob, or
1 12-ounce can white corn, drained
6 pimiento-stuffed green olives, chopped
8 black olives, chopped
½ tablespoon chili powder
½ teaspoon cumin
¼ teaspoon cayenne
¼ cup currants or raisins
1 tablespoon instant minced onion
2 tablespoons oil
1 cup or 1 10-ounce can beef gravy
½ cup sherry (optional)
Hi-Fiber Pastry for 1-crust pie

Combine all ingredients but crust; place in greased round casserole. (Those who prefer not to use sherry may use ¼ cup of orange juice and ¼ cup of water instead.) Prepare pastry, roll out to fit top of casserole, cutting slits in center; lay over filling. Bake in preheated hot oven (400–425° F.) until crust is browned and filling bubbling. Makes 4–6 servings.

Note: For those to whom rolling out pie crust seems the most formidable of tasks, a frozen ready-to-use crust may be substituted, but to make up for the fiber lack, add 2 tablespoons of bran meal to the sauce for the filling, plus another 2 tablespoons of liquid. When baked, the bran is completely dissolved in the sauce.

Tuna Pie with Oat Biscuit Crust

FILLING:

1 large can (15 ounce) or 2 6- or 7-ounce cans chunk-style tuna, drained
1 teaspoon grated lemon rind
2 tablespoons minced parsley
½ cup diced briefly cooked carrots
1 10½-ounce can condensed cream of mushroom soup
1 cup light cream or whole milk

CRUST:

¾ cup buckwheat or whole-wheat pancake mix
¼ cup rolled oats
3 tablespoons shortening
¼ cup milk

To drained tuna, add remaining ingredients in order given. Place filling in greased 1½-quart casserole.

To make crust, combine pancake mix and oats; cut in shortening. Stir in milk just until dry ingredients are moistened and dough can be worked into a ball. Roll out on lightly floured surface to fit top of casserole. Cut 3 slashes in center. Place loosely over filling (it need not be sealed to rim). Bake in hot oven preheated to 425° F. until crust is golden and sauce bubbling (about 35 minutes). Makes 4–6 servings.

Note: If preferred, make ½ recipe 100 Percent Whole-Wheat Pancake batter (see recipe, page 53), add oats, shortening, and milk.

Beef and Vegetable Pie

Hi-Fiber Pastry for 1-crust
  pie
1½ cups diced cooked beef
  (leftover roast)
1 10-ounce package frozen
  peas and carrots
1 10-ounce package frozen
  baby butter beans
2 tablespoons minced
  parsley

1 tablespoon instant minced
  onion
½ teaspoon salt
¼ teaspoon seasoned salt
1¼ cups beef bouillon
4 tablespoons crushed
  whole-bran cereal or bran
  meal
1 tablespoon sherry
  (optional)

Prepare pastry; roll out to fit top of round casserole; cut slits
in center. Combine remaining ingredients for filling (soak the
bran in beef bouillon separately, for about 3 minutes, before
adding to other ingredients). Frozen vegetables need not be
precooked. Place beef and vegetable mixture in casserole, top
with crust. Bake in hot oven (400° F.) for 30–40 minutes,
or until crust is golden and filling bubbling beneath it. Makes
4 servings.

Golubtsi
(Russian Stuffed Cabbage)

12 large cabbage leaves
Salt
  1 medium onion, chopped
  4 tablespoons butter
  2 tablespoons minced
    parsley
1½ cups coarse crumbs of
    dark rye bread
  ¾ pound ground lean pork

or beef
1 egg, beaten
1½ cups canned pureed
    tomatoes or tomato sauce
2 tablespoons whole-bran
    cereal
½ cup water
½ cup sour cream or plain
    yogurt

Separate outer cabbage leaves carefully; cut away hard core.
Place leaves in deep pot, cover with *boiling* water, and sprinkle
with salt; cook for 2 minutes, let stand in water for 10 minutes, then drain well.

Meantime, simmer onion in 2 tablespoons of butter until yellowed; add parsley, breadcrumbs, meat, and salt; cook until meat has lost its pink color. Cool. Stir in egg and 1 tablespoon of tomato puree or sauce. Season to taste. Remove cabbage leaves, place on board, and spoon 1–1½ tablespoons of meat mixture inside each leaf. Fold over ends, then sides, and roll up tightly. Melt remaining butter and brush over bottom of shallow casserole. Place rolled cabbage leaves in casserole, overlapped side down. Simmer in butter on top of stove over very low heat for 2 minutes. (For those concerned about keeping fat intake down, this step may be omitted.) Soften bran in water; add to this the remaining tomato puree or sauce, and pour over cabbage rolls. Bake covered (use foil if casserole has no cover) in moderate oven (350° F.) for 1 hour. Spoon sour cream or yogurt over top shortly before removing from oven. Serve with baked potatoes or potatoes boiled in their jackets. Serves 6.

Vegetarian Stuffed Cabbage

12 large cabbage leaves
2 cups cooked millet or bulgur, or Wheatena
1 cup chopped peanuts
½ cup diced celery
¼ cup grated raw carrots
¼ cup minced onion
¼ cup currants or raisins

½ teaspoon salt
2 tablespoons soy sauce
1 cup beef bouillon
2 tablespoons tomato paste
1 tablespoon whole-bran cereal
Yogurt

Blanche cabbage leaves with boiling water as described in previous recipe. Combine remaining ingredients (except bouillon, tomato paste, bran, and yogurt). Season to taste. Divide mixture among cabbage leaves and roll up, as in the previous recipe. Arrange cabbage rolls in bottom of shallow casserole. Combine beef bouillon, tomato paste, and bran; let stand until bran is softened and dissolved. Pour over cabbage rolls. Bake covered in moderate (350° F.) oven for 20 minutes, or until sauce is bubbling; uncover, bake 10–15 minutes longer, until cabbage is soft. Spoon a little of sauce over cabbage rolls. Serve with yogurt as a separate sauce. Makes 6 servings.

Boston Baked Beans

1 quart (4 cups) navy or pea beans
½ pound salt pork, cut in small cubes
3 or 4 tablespoons molasses
1 cup water

1 teaspoon prepared mustard
¼ teaspoon powdered ginger
1 tablespoon catsup

Soak beans overnight; drain, cover with fresh water, heat slowly (do not boil) until the skins burst. (Test a bean or two by taking out in a spoon and blow on it—the skins will burst if they are ready.) Drain beans once more. Place about half the pork in a deep earthenware casserole or bean-pot. Heat together remaining ingredients, add to cooked drained beans, pour over salt pork in pot. Place remaining chunks of pork in the beans, with 2 or 3 large pieces on top. Add enough water to barely cover. Put cover on casserole or bean-pot, bake for 6–8 hours in a very slow oven (200° F.). It may be necessary to add more water; take a look now and then to see. Makes about 8 servings.

Vegetarian Boston Beans

Omit salt pork, add ½ pound of Morningstar or other vegetable protein sausages. Otherwise, prepare exactly the same way as in recipe above.

Boston Brown Bread and Indian Pudding are traditionally served with baked beans. All three dishes are exceptionally high in fiber. In olden days there was a big black cast-iron stove in every kitchen, and during the winter the stove was used not only for cooking, but to heat the kitchen as well, bringing the family together there for warmth. So the casseroles baking in the oven and bread steaming away in a kettle on the stove served a double purpose. We had such a stove in our kitchen when I was a child, and these three dishes were our wintertime favorites. I recommend them all. (For Indian Pudding, made the old-fashioned way, see Chapter 13.)

Cholent

In Orthodox Jewish homes, no cooking is permitted on the Sabbath (Saturday), so long-cooking casseroles are often begun on Friday night—just as the Pilgrim Fathers baked their beans all night on Saturday since *they* permitted no cooking in the home on Sunday.

For best results, this should be slow-baked in an oven, or it can be cooked in a crock-pot for at least 12 hours.

2 cups fava or dried lima
  beans
2 pounds brisket of beef,
  carefully trimmed of all fat
3 tablespoons chicken fat
3 onions, coarsely chopped
2 garlic cloves, minced

2 teaspoons salt
¼ teaspoon black pepper
¼ teaspoon powdered ginger
1 cup buckwheat groats
  (kasha) or millet
2 teaspoons paprika
Boiling water as needed

Soak dried beans for 12 hours before cooking; drain. Sear meat in chicken fat over high heat in large deep pot (or crock-pot). Add onion, garlic, and seasonings; cook until lightly browned. Add drained beans and the kasha or millet. Add *boiling* water enough to rise 1 inch above beans. Cover tightly; if using an earthenware pot, seal with flour paste around edges of cover. Bake 12 hours at 300° F. or 24 hours at 250° F.

Chili con Carne

2 tablespoons oil or
  shortening
2 garlic cloves
2 or 3 large onions, sliced
½ green pepper, seeded and
  chopped
1 tablespoon chili powder
½ teaspoon cumin
½ teaspoon oregano

Cayenne or Tabasco sauce to
  taste
½–¾ pound ground beef
1-pound can tomatoes, or 1
  8-ounce can tomato sauce
1-pound can red kidney beans
1 cup water or broth
Salt to taste

Heat oil, add garlic, cook until yellow and soft, then crush into the oil. Add onion, stir-fry over moderate heat until lightly browned. Add green pepper, chili powder, and other seasonings, stir to blend. Add meat (a cheap grade of ground beef may be used), cook until it loses its pink color. Add tomatoes and kidney beans with their liquid, water, and salt. Simmer, covered, about 40 minutes. This dish may be served immediately but is better if cooked ahead, chilled (so that fat will rise to top and can be skimmed), then reheated. Serve with rice or millet and a green salad. Makes 6 servings.

Vegetarian Tamale Pie

Prepare Chili con Carne as above, but omit meat; either double the amount of kidney beans, or use 2 cups of cooked rice plus the beans. Place chili in a large casserole, cover with the following mixture, and bake until crust is browned.

1 cup stone-ground yellow cornmeal or masa	¼ cup cold water
	1 egg, beaten
½ teaspoon baking soda	½ cup buttermilk
½ teaspoon salt	

Combine cornmeal, baking soda, and salt; add water, let stand for 5 minutes. Then add egg and buttermilk. Spoon batter over top of chili. Bake about 40 minutes. Makes 6–8 servings.

Millet Nut Casserole

½ cup raisins or currants	1 cup mixed chopped nuts
⅓ cup chopped dried apricots	2 tablespoons melted butter
Cold water to cover	or margarine
2 cups *cooked* millet	

Soak fruit in water to cover for ½ hour; drain (save liquid for sweetening to use in bread dough or puddings). Combine cooked millet with nuts and fruit, place in greased 1-quart casserole. Brush melted butter over top. Serve warm with cooked collard greens and broiled or baked tomatoes. Makes 6 servings as an entree, or can be served as a side dish. (Any combination of nuts may be used, including sunflower kernels, toasted soybeans, and roasted chestnuts.)

In the north of India, curries are milder and sweeter than in the southern subtropical areas. By mixing one's own selection of spices, it is possible to come up with a delicious curry mixture that is not so hot it takes off the top of your head!

Eggplant Curry

(LC)

1 medium onion, thinly sliced
2 garlic cloves, crushed
4 tablespoons oil
1 green pepper, cut in chunks
1 teaspoon Madras curry powder
½ teaspoon turmeric or dry mustard
1 teaspoon cumin
½ teaspoon allspice
¼ teaspoon cayenne
½ teaspoon Szechuan pepper (optional)
½ teaspoon salt, or to taste

3 cups diced (unpeeled) eggplant
¼ cup currants or raisins
1 cup fresh green peas or tender snap beans
1 apple, pared and chopped
1 large or 2 small carrots, cut in thin sticks
1 cup water
½ cup dry-roasted peanuts or toasted soybeans
¼ cup shredded coconut
Yogurt
Chutney

Stir-fry onion and garlic in 2 tablespoons of oil until soft; add the green pepper, spices, and salt, and cook for 30 seconds longer. Push onion to one side of pan, remove green pepper. Add more oil and the eggplant. Stir-fry eggplant until well moistened, moving almost continuously. Add fruit, peas or beans, carrots, and water. Simmer at low heat *uncovered* until all vegetables are tender (about 8–10 minutes). (The apple should cook to a mush, thickening the sauce.) Replace green pepper, add nuts, and cook for 1 minute longer. Serve sprinkled with coconut. Pass yogurt and chutney (see following recipe). Makes about 6 servings.

Quick Chutney

1 cup apricot, peach, or
  plum jam
½ teaspoon curry powder
¼ teaspoon powdered
  mustard or turmeric
¼ teaspoon cumin

⅓ cup chopped nuts
1 teaspoon vinegar or lemon
  juice
2 chopped soft-type pitted
  prunes, cut in half

Combine all ingredients, blend well, heat just to point of boiling, then remove from stove. Serve cold. If a spicier chutney is preferred, add more curry powder. Makes about 1½ cups.

Vegetarian Chow Mein

(LC)

¼ cup oil (approx.)
½ cup thinly sliced onion
2 garlic cloves
1 cup fresh or frozen green
  peas
½ cup bok choy or celery
  cabbage, cut in 2-inch
  pieces, or cauliflower
  leaves
½ cup green pepper in chunks
1 cup fresh cauliflower,
  broken in small pieces
Fresh bean sprouts (optional)

1 cup bamboo shoots
4 or 5 water chestnuts, sliced
1 cup peanuts or toasted
  soybeans
2 tablespoons soy flour
2–3 tablespoons soy sauce
½ teaspoon salt
1 tablespoon sherry
  (optional)
½ cup water or broth
Sautéed Wheat Chex for
  topping

Heat 2 tablespoons of oil in wok or deep heavy skillet. Add onion and garlic; cook until golden (about 2 minutes). Press garlic cloves into oil with tines of fork (remove shreds). Add peas, cook for 2 minutes; add bok choy, or celery cabbage, and green pepper, cook for 1 or 2 minutes longer. Remove all these with slotted spoon to a bowl. Add more oil if necessary. Add cauliflower, cook for 2–3 minutes. Add bean sprouts and bamboo shoots, cook just to heat through. Replace previously cooked vegetables, add water chestnuts and nuts or soybeans. Add to soy flour the soy sauce, salt, and sherry to form a paste. Stir into this water or broth, then add to vegetables and cook, stirring, until sauce is thickened (about 3 minutes). Serve topped with the Wheat Chex rather than fried noodles. (Or prepare your own fried noodles with whole-wheat noodles from a health store, as suggested on page 36.) Makes 4–6 servings.

Variations: Add soaked black mushrooms or lily buds; use boiled chestnuts rather than water chestnuts; broccoli, cut into small pieces, instead of cauliflower; or snow peas instead of green peas.

Bok choy, if it can be found, makes a delightful addition to any Chinese entree. Look for it in Oriental groceries.

Fried Brown Rice

1 tablespoon butter or margarine	½ teaspoon salt
1 tablespoon oil	½ pound very thin slices of beef or pork, cut in strips
1 medium onion, chopped	2 cups *cooked* brown rice
1 small yellow squash (3 inches), thinly sliced, not peeled	¼ cup slivered almonds
	1–2 tablespoons soy sauce
½ cup diced green pepper	1 egg beaten with 2 tablespoons water

Melt butter or margarine with oil in skillet; add onion, cook until lightly browned. Add squash, green pepper, and salt; stir-fry for 60 seconds; remove. Add meat, stir-fry about 2 minutes. Add rice, stir to blend. Replace vegetables, add nuts and soy sauce, then quickly stir in egg-water mixture, stirring constantly so that egg is blended with rice completely. (There should be no visible bits of egg white.) Serve immediately. Makes 3 or 4 single-entree servings.

Vegetarian Brown Rice

Instead of meat, add 2 cups of cooked or canned chickpeas or red kidney beans.

Baked Stuffed Vegetarian Peppers

4 large well-shaped green
  peppers
3 tablespoons oil
1 or 2 garlic cloves
2 cups slightly stale whole-
  grain bread, broken in
  small pieces
¼ cup dried currants

½ cup sunflower kernels or
  coarsely crushed toasted
  soybeans
½ teaspoon thyme
¼ teaspoon salt
Dash of cayenne
¼ cup grated Parmesan
  cheese

Trim and seed peppers, leaving them whole but removing all white membrane and seeds. See if they will stand up steadily; if not, cut a very thin slice from the bottoms of those that seem wobbly. Pour *boiling* water over peppers, let stand about 2 minutes in water, then drain well, while preparing filling.

Place oil in skillet, add garlic, cook until soft, then press garlic into the oil to release the juices. (The garlic may then be discarded—it has left that "suspicion" of flavor.) Add the bread, sauté in the oil until lightly browned. Add fruit, sunflower kernels or soybeans, and thyme. Remove stuffing to bowl; add salt and cayenne to taste.

Brush drained peppers with olive oil inside and out. Fill with the stuffing. Place close together in a baking dish. Top each with cheese. Bake in a moderate oven (350° F.) for 45 minutes to an hour until peppers are soft. Halfway through the baking period, brush with additional oil. Serves 4.

Vegetarian Lasagne

½ pound whole-wheat
  lasagne noodles
¼ cup chopped onion
¼ cup chopped parsley
2 tablespoons chopped
  pimiento
¼ cup chopped green pepper
2 garlic cloves, crushed
3 tablespoons olive oil
1 large can (1 pound 12
  ounces) plum tomatoes
1 6-ounce can tomato paste
1 teaspoon oregano
½ teaspoon dried basil, or
  1 tablespoon chopped
  fresh basil

½ teaspoon salt, or to taste
1 10-ounce package frozen
  mixed vegetables
½ cup chopped celery
½ cup sunflower kernels or
  toasted slivered almonds
1 pound (16 ounces)
  creamed cottage cheese
  or ricotta cheese
½ cup grated Parmesan
  cheese
½ pound (8 ounces) moz-
  zarella cheese
½ cup crushed Wheat Chex
  or 40% Bran

Cook noodles; drain, cut to measure baking dish.

Sauté onion, parsley, pimiento, green pepper, and garlic in olive oil until soft. Add canned tomatoes and tomato paste, herbs, and salt. Simmer for 15 minutes. Add frozen vegetables and celery; continue to cook about 5 minutes. Stir in nuts.

Arrange cooked noodles in layers with the sauce, adding cottage cheese or ricotta, Parmesan, and slices of mozzarella over each layer. The tomato mixture and mozzarella should be on top. Sprinkle crushed cereal over mozzarella. Bake in moderate oven (350–375° F.) until cheese is melted and sauce bubbling (about ½ hour). Makes 10 servings.

Baked Dried Lima Casserole

2 cups dried lima beans
1 garlic clove, minced
1 medium onion, chopped
1 medium carrot, pared,
  grated
2 tablespoons butter or
  margarine
¼ cup minced parsley

1 cup tomato juice
Water
Salt, pepper
½ cup shredded Swiss cheese
½ cup finely crushed
  Shredded Wheat or
  Triscuits

Soak limas the night before; drain. Cook garlic, onion, and carrot in butter until lightly browned; add parsley. Add to beans with tomato juice and water to come to ½ inch above level of beans. Cover tightly, simmer over low heat about 2 hours, adding more water as needed. (If cooked in a crockpot, add water to 1 inch above beans, cook all day at very low heat.) Transfer to 1½-quart casserole, top with mixture of cheese and crushed cereal. Bake in moderately hot oven until cheese is melted. (If beans are hot when placed in casserole, simply put cereal and cheese over top and slip under broiler.) Makes 6–8 servings.

Creole Baked Stuffed Eggplant

(LC)

1 medium-to-large eggplant
1 medium onion, chopped
1 green pepper, seeded and chopped
½ cup diced celery
2 tablespoons oil
2 large or 3 smaller tomatoes, chopped
1 teaspoon salt
½ bay leaf, crumbled
2 tablespoons chopped pecans or walnuts
Pinch of cloves
Pinch of cayenne
2 cups crumbled whole-wheat bread
½ cup grated cheese
Butter

Carefully remove stem of eggplant; slice lengthwise, then scoop out eggplant, leaving a boat shape. Brush all over with oil or melted butter or margarine; sprinkle with salt.

Sauté onion, green pepper, and celery in oil until lightly browned. Add tomato, salt, and bay leaf. Cook about 5 minutes. Add nuts, cloves, cayenne, and breadcrumbs. Place in hollowed eggplant, with the chopped-up eggplant pulp removed from the inside. Over the top spread grated cheese. Dot generously with butter. Bake in a moderately hot oven (375° F.) about 1 hour, or until eggplant is completely tender. Makes 4–6 servings.

CHAPTER 10

Vegetables and
Other Side Dishes

Of all high-fiber foods, vegetables are lowest in calories and therefore of special interest for weight control. Some consider vegetables more effective as fiber when they are served raw (for relishes and in salads) rather than cooked. If cooked, the timing should be very brief—except for limas, which need thorough cooking to be easily digested.

Try to buy vegetables at the peak of season locally—they lose flavor and food value during storage and transportation. The fiber content of frozen vegetables is the same as fresh, except that transportation and storage can impair flavor and cause loss of vitamins when the frozen food undergoes alternate thawing and refreezing.

Use seeds and herbs for flavor in vegetable cookery and to gain fiber, too. Both fresh coriander leaves and parsley have twice as much fiber *per pound* as spinach. Parsley may be used in very large quantities; it's one of the few seasoners that does not overpower other flavors, yet adds piquancy.

Fresh coriander is still unknown in most parts of the country, but it has a promising future. Look for it in Latin-American, Oriental, East-Indian, and Armenian groceries. The Arabian name for it is kizbara, the Latinos call it cilantro or culantro, the Portuguese call it coentro, in Oriental markets it is "Chinese parsley" or what sounds to me like *im-sayh*.

ALPHABETICAL GUIDE TO
VEGETABLE COOKERY

Artichokes. Whole fresh artichokes: cut off stem and tips of leaves, remove tough outer leaves. Place on rack in kettle with salted water, lemon juice, a spoonful of olive oil. Cook with cover slightly ajar for 30–40 minutes, or until tender; test by inserting point of sharp knife in stem. Drain thoroughly; work choke of each loose by scooping out with a spoon. Serve whole with individual bowls of lemon butter for dipping. (*Lemon Butter:* Heat together 4 tablespoons of butter, 1 tablespoon of lemon juice, just until butter melts.)

Artichoke Bottoms. The most tender part, with all leaves removed.

Baby Artichokes. When very small, lay artichokes on sides in saucepan, cook in boiling salted water for 10–15 minutes, or until fork-tender. Cut in quarters. (These are "artichoke hearts.")

Frozen Artichoke Hearts. Cook according to package directions but use olive oil (only) instead of water, and add a garlic clove. When cooked, sprinkle with lemon juice.

Artichokes à la Polita

(LC)

12 baby artichokes, or 10-ounce package artichoke hearts	2 cups water
10 small white onions	1 teaspoon salt
1 small carrot, cubed	1 tablespoon minced parsley or mint
½ cup olive oil	2 tablespoons lemon juice
	1 teaspoon cornstarch

Prepare artichokes as described above; if large, quarter, then cut away choke. If small, leave whole. Brown onion and carrot in oil in heavy saucepan, turning occasionally. Add water, salt, parsley or mint, artichokes, and lemon juice. Simmer partially covered for 15 minutes, or until fork will penetrate stem of largest artichoke. Remove vegetables. Dissolve cornstarch in cold water, add to hot liquid, simmer until thickened. Replace vegetables in sauce. Serve at room temperature, not chilled, as an hors d'oeuvres or buffet offering.

Asparagus. When purchasing, examine tips of spears: if withered, the vegetable was picked some time ago. Clean by holding spears under running water, brush with stiff vegetable brush, then take each spear in your hands and bend it backward. The spear will break at the the point where the stem begins to toughen. (No amount of cooking will make the lower stem edible.) Lay spears flat in frying pan; add salted water barely to cover, place lid over pan at an angle so steam may escape. Cook 5–7 minutes until a fork can be plunged into largest spear easily. Drain; save liquid for soup. Add a dab of butter immediately if it is to be served warm; marinate while warm in Oil-Vinegar Dressing if it is to be served cold.

Asparagus on Toast. For lunch, serve spears over whole-wheat toast, dribble a teaspoon of cooking liquid over toast, dot with butter.

Asparagus Vinaigrette. Marinate cooked or canned spears in Oil-Vinegar Dressing, and serve topped with crumbled egg yolk and/or bacon bits.

Beet Greens. Select beets with fresh green leaves and you get two vegetables for the price of one. Put beet roots away for a later meal, trim leaves, cutting off stems. Cook leaves in a moderate amount of salted water, covered, until tender (about 10 minutes). Drain thoroughly; dress while warm with oil and vinegar or butter and lemon juice.

Beets (*Beet Root*). Cook whole *without peeling* in boiling salted water, covered, until fork-tender. Cooking time varies according to size and maturity of beets. When tender, drain, cool until easily handled, then peel off skin, reheat in butter or in oil and vinegar (or lemon juice). If small, serve whole. If large, slice or dice.

Beets with Caraway. Add about 1 teaspoon of caraway seeds to butter when reheating beets.

Beets with Sour Cream or Yogurt. Serve cooked or canned beets with sauce of sour cream or yogurt to which chopped parsley or freeze-dried chives have been added. Delicious hot as a vegetable, cold as an hors d'oeuvres (serve small whole beets around sauce for dipping).

Beets with Bran or Wheat Germ. When reheating, add a spoonful of whole-bran cereal or Kretchmer wheat germ to beets in butter.

Beets Vinaigrette. Marinate cooked beets in Oil-Vinegar Dressing or Vinaigrette Dressing. Good both hot and cold.

Black-Eyed Peas. Frozen black-eyed peas are immature (green) peas which require only about 12 minutes cooking. Dried black-eyed peas (also called cowpeas) must be presoaked and require hours of cooking. The traditional Southern dish always served on New Year's Day may be made with either. (When rice is added, it becomes Hopping John.)

Southern-Style Black-Eyed Peas

2 pounds fresh shelled black-
   eyed peas
Water, salt
1 onion, chopped
½ cup chopped green pepper

1 celery stalk, chopped
1 can (1 pound) tomatoes
Bits of chopped ham or bacon
Seasonings to taste

Put shelled peas in heavy saucepan with remaining ingredients, simmer covered until peas are tender (cooking time varies with maturity of peas when picked). Makes 10 servings.

Dried Black-Eyed Peas. Soak 1 pound of peas overnight; drain, place in pan with 2 quarts of water and remaining ingredients as given above; simmer about 2 hours, or until tender.

Bok Choy. Look for this in markets catering to Americans of Oriental background or in Chinese markets. It looks like a cauliflower which failed to head and the leaves have a flavor somewhat like cooked cauliflower leaves, but spicier. Used primarily as one of the vegetables in Chinese entrees, cut in 2-inch lengths, stir-fried.

Broccoli. Separate into individual spears, cut off tougher portion of stems, also leaves, if desired. (But slivered stem and leaves may be cooked as a separate vegetable.) If cut into small pieces, broccoli will cook in about 8 minutes; first heat salted water to boiling, add broccoli, cook with lid partially ajar. When tender, drain, add butter and lemon juice. (It cannot be reheated successfully, but leftovers can be used in making Eggs or Chicken Divan.)

Chinese-Style Broccoli. Cook short, slivered spears in oil rather than water for 2–3 minutes, stirring to avoid scorching. Remove, sprinkle with slivered toasted almonds. (If combined with other vegetables and meat or fish, first cook broccoli, remove, replace during last few minutes of cooking.)

Brussels Sprouts. Trim only stem end, add to boiling salted water, keeping lid slightly ajar as they cook (to allow steam to escape and retain bright color), and cook only until barely tender (4–5 minutes). Test with a fork for doneness. (Useless as leftovers; never add sprouts to a stew, they will destroy it.)

Butter Beans. A Southern name for lima beans that are allowed to become more mature before harvesting, they are therefore less tender than regular limas and require longer cooking time.

Cabbage, Green or White. To serve as a hot vegetable, cut in slices ⅛- to ¼-inch thick; cook in small amount of salted water just until wilted and fork-tender (7–8 minutes). Drain thoroughly, dress with butter or margarine and lemon juice.

With Yogurt-Ginger Sauce. Instead of butter, add plain yogurt (or sour cream) and a dash of powdered ginger; toss cabbage to coat well.

Cabbage with Peanuts. Shred cabbage but bake in a casserole: to 1 quart of shredded cabbage, add ⅓ cup of chopped peanuts, ½ teaspoon of salt, and 2 tablespoons of milk (no water). Bake covered for ½ hour.

Carrots. The briefer the cooking, the more flavorful the carrots. Scrape, cut lengthwise in halves or quarters (depending on size), then cut each in half again. Or slice thinly crosswise. Cook tightly covered with ½ cup of water, ¼ teaspoon of salt, until barely fork-tender (about 4 minutes); drain. Or steam on vegetable rack. Add butter and chopped parsley or other seasoning, while warm.

With Orange Nut Sauce. Cook carrots in orange juice instead of water, add salt as usual. When tender, remove from saucepan, add ½ teaspoon of honey to remaining orange juice, cook until juice is reduced and thickened. Pour syrup over carrots, sprinkle with chopped peanuts or toasted slivered almonds.

Caraway Carrots. Slice carrots lengthwise in quarters; cook briefly, drain, add ½ tablespoon of caraway seeds (for 4 large carrots), 1 tablespoon of butter, and 2 tablespoons of chopped parsley.

(See also Spiced Carrots and Mushrooms, page 37.)

Carrots and Cauliflower. Dice carrots; break cauliflower into small buds. Cook separately until tender. Serve together in same dish, dressed with butter, sprinkled with parsley, chopped fresh coriander, or chopped dill, and toasted sesame seeds.

Cauliflower. Before cooking, remove leaves (save tender leaves to cook as a separate vegetable or in a Chinese entree). Cut into small buds for quicker cooking, or keep whole if preferred for appearance. Bathe with butter, sprinkle with paprika; serve with lemon wedges.

Cauliflower with Coriander. Add chopped fresh coriander or crushed coriander seeds to cooked cauliflower.

With Cheese Sauce. As cauliflower cooks, make a quick sauce by combining ½ can of condensed Cheddar soup with milk to desired consistency; heat until bubbling. Pour over whole cooked cauliflower.

Bran-Crowned Cauliflower. Melt 2 tablespoons of butter, stir in 3 tablespoons of whole-bran cereal or Kretchmer wheat germ. Add to cooked cauliflower (broken into buds), stir to distribute.

Celeriac or Celery Root. A big brown knob, about the same size as rutabaga, the only obvious relation this bears to Pascal celery is in the leaves which may be so wilted they've been broken off. Pare off rind, cut root into sticks. The French usually serve it raw, the Germans cook it and add a cream sauce. Raw, it makes a crunchy hors d'oeuvres; creamed, it is a nice side dish.

Celery or Pascal Celery. Useful both raw as a salad ingredient or appetizer and cooked as a vegetable. Slice at an angle into 2-inch pieces, cook in salted water until tender (10–12 minutes), dress with butter and lemon juice. Add toasted sesame seeds, if desired.

Celery in Tomato Sauce. Instead of water, cook celery in tomato juice or chopped tomato (enough just to cover) with some thinly sliced onion and salt. When celery is tender, increase heat to reduce and thicken sauce. Serve topped with minced parsley or dill.

Celery in Chicken Broth. Instead of water and salt, cook in chicken broth made with concentrate or cubes; when tender, drain, sprinkle with fennel or anise seeds and butter. (Save broth for soup or gravy.)

Celery in Orange Juice. Instead of water, cook in orange juice (salted) with a little thyme and a pinch of powdered ginger.

Celery Cabbage. This elongated member of the cabbage family is good both raw (in a salad or as a dip for spreads) and cooked. It is most often used as an ingredient in Chinese entrees, but is also cooked in any of the ways suggested for celery above.

Chard, or Swiss Chard. The white part of the leaves requires longer cooking than the green tops so cut separately, cook white part first, for 5 minutes, before adding green. Dress simply with oil and vinegar or follow Spinach Catalan recipe but allow longer cooking time.

Collards. An excellent source not only of fiber but also of calcium, potassium, and Vitamin A, these greens should be served more often. To cook, remove tough outer part of stem, chop stems and leaves in small pieces. For 1 quart, add 1 cup of water, ½ teaspoon of salt, and cook until tender (about 10 minutes). Drain thoroughly. Dress with oil and vinegar or with butter. Also good as a cold cooked salad.

Collards Catalan. Follow recipe for Spinach Catalan, substituting collards for spinach; allow longer cooking time.

Frozen collard greens have same fiber, vitamin, and mineral content as fresh and require only brief cooking (about 4 minutes).

Corn on Cob. Fresh or frozen sweet corn has more fiber than any other corn product. Place ears in, or on rack above, salted water already boiling hard, cook covered about 6 minutes. Or cook in pressure cooker about 2 minutes. Will be easier to chew and will relinquish more of its natural sweetness if, before serving (when cooked), it is cut lengthwise through center of kernels with sharp knife, then buttered.

Succotash. Before cooking, cut lengthwise through rows of kernels, then scrape off kernels into saucepan. Cook corn in 2 tablespoons each of butter and water over low heat, tightly covered, for 3 minutes. Add about same quantity *cooked* lima, snap beans, or broadbeans, cook 2–3 minutes longer. Season with salt and black pepper; add cream, if desired.

Dandelion Greens. Rarely sold in the markets, they are plentiful in early spring in yards or along roadways. Cook briefly in salted water, add oil and vinegar or butter and lemon juice. An excellent source of fiber, calcium, and Vitamin A, dandelion greens are very low in calories. Also good raw in salads.

Eggplant. A good fiber source, useful for entrees and as a side dish. Do not peel: the peel adds flavor. The small so-called Italian eggplants are more tender, less likely to be bitter, and a good choice for small households. Select those entirely free from bruised or soft spots; better slightly green than overripe.

Slice lengthwise, crosswise, or cut in cubes. Flavor is best with olive oil, but it soaks up oil like a sponge. Mediterranean cooks sprinkle each slice with salt, let stand for 10–15 minutes, then rinse; supposedly this makes eggplant less bitter and prevents some absorption of oil.

The quickest way to prepare it as a side dish is to cut it in small pieces, stir-fry in oil almost constantly until lightly browned, and sprinkle with salt as it cooks. Serve topped with chopped parsley.

Charcoal-Broiled Eggplant Kabobs. Cut eggplant in ¾-inch cubes; marinate in a mixture of olive oil, juice, salt, and oregano, turning several times until well moistened. Spear on barbecue skewers, brown over charcoal, turning frequently. If desired, alternate eggplant with green pepper squares and yellow summer squash (also marinated).

Baked Eggplant Slices

8 ¼-inch eggplant slices	½ teaspoon salt
3 tablespoons olive oil (approx.)	¼ cup finely crushed Shredded Wheat
Salt, pepper	¼ cup chopped parsley
3 tablespoons soy flour	

Cut large eggplant crosswise (save unused portion, plastic-wrap for another meal), brush each side with oil, then dust with salt, pepper, and flour. Place in one layer in large shallow roasting pan or baking sheet. Place in oven preheated to 375° F., bake for 10 minutes. Turn, sprinkle with mixture of Shredded Wheat and parsley; add more oil. Bake until crumb topping is browned and eggplant tender (about 5 minutes more). Serves 4.

Fennel. This curious-looking vegetable with bulbous root and feathery top has a decided licorice flavor. Cook the root like celery; use the top, chopped, as an herb for salads, hard-cooked eggs, and sandwich fillings.

Green Beans. Not as high in fiber as limas but a good fiber source and lowest in calories of all legumes, green or dried. In early summer, when very tender and small, they're good raw; they require no more than 7 minutes to cook. When slightly older and more plump, slice lengthwise (frenched), then cut again in half; can be cooked in less than 5 minutes. To serve hot, add butter; for Green Beans Vinaigrette, add oil and vinegar while warm.

Cumin-Flavored Beans. Stir-fry tender young snap beans with thin-sliced scallions in oil or butter; sprinkle with salt and crushed cumin, serve hot.

Greek-Style Beans in Tomato Sauce. Use beans that were quite mature when picked: break into pieces, place in heavy saucepan with fully ripe tomatoes (skinned and chopped), sliced onions, 1 or 2 minced garlic cloves, and a generous quantity of olive oil—but *no* water. Season with salt and oregano to taste. Simmer covered over low heat until fork-tender (cooking time depends on tenderness of beans). Excellent with a barbecue meal, good cold or hot.

Greek-Style Limas and *Greek-Style Wax Beans* can be cooked the same way, substituting limas or wax beans for the green beans.

Green beans are also delicious with slivered almonds or sliced mushrooms or with diced red sweet pepper.

Green Peas. When fresh out of the home garden, peas are divine: they need only 10 minutes cooking, have exquisite flavor, need no other embellishment but butter. But supermarket fresh peas are always a gamble; the bigger the peas inside the pod, the more cooking they need and the less flavor they furnish.

Frozen peas are better if cooked in butter and only 2 tablespoons of water than just plain boiled; season with salt, powdered fennel, crushed mint, *or* chopped fresh dill.

Petit Pois à la Française

1 small head Boston lettuce	1 teaspoon sugar
3 pounds peas in pod (or 1-pound can early spring peas)	½ teaspoon salt
	4 tablespoons butter
	Pinch of nutmeg
3 tablespoons minced shallot or scallion	¼ cup water
	1 tablespoon minced parsley

Place a layer of shredded lettuce in a saucepan with a tight-fitting lid; add shelled peas and 3–4 pods. Add all remaining ingredients but parsley; cover with remaining lettuce. Cover tightly, bring to a boil, lower heat, cook for 12–15 minutes until peas are all wrinkled. Shake pan now and then to prevent sticking. Remove, discard lettuce and pods. Serve sprinkled with parsley. Makes 6 servings.

Italian Beans or Broadbeans. The frozen "Italian" beans are among the most satisfactory of the frozen vegetables; cook as directed. Fresh green broadbeans are a variety of pole beans, very long, very wide. Cook by any of the variations suggested for Green Beans.

Kale. Cook exactly like Collards.

Lima Beans. Highest in fiber of any fresh vegetables, but also highest in calories (except for sweet potatoes). Allow plenty of cooking time—15–20 minutes for fresh limas. If under-cooked, they are difficult to digest. Frozen limas, both the Fordhook and baby limas, are generally a more economical buy than the fresh, and if you're lucky, you may get some with full flavor, too. See Succotash (under *Corn*), Greek-Style Beans in Tomato Sauce, and entrees using limas.

Mushrooms. Always wash fresh mushrooms thoroughly before cooking (but not before storing—water hastens their wilting), but do not peel; trim woodier portion of stems.

Sautéed in Butter. Slice, stir-fry (2 tablespoons of butter for ¼ pound of mushrooms) until nicely browned; sprinkle with salt.

Creamed Mushrooms. Sauté either crowns or sliced mushrooms in butter until lightly browned, then add same amount of whole-wheat or soy flour as butter, slowly stir in 1 cup of milk for each 2 tablespoons of butter and flour; simmer until thickened.

Okra. My favorite way of cooking okra is a trick I learned from a Southerner, Nona Wegner. Cut pods crosswise into ½-inch slices, stir-fry in oil, margarine, or butter for about 2–3 minutes until fork-tender but still crisp. Serve sprinkled with lemon juice. Quick, easy, delicious!

Mediterranean Okra. Cook 1 cup of sliced onion and a minced garlic clove in 2 tablespoons of olive oil until golden but not browned; add 2 cups of tomato juice, salt, pepper, and a pinch of thyme. Simmer for 5 minutes until reduced; add 1 teaspoon of fresh lemon juice and grated rind. Add either fresh (1½ cups) or frozen okra (10-ounce package), and continue to cook *uncovered* until okra is tender but still bright green.

Onions. When a recipe specifies *cooking onion in oil* (or butter or other fat), the heat should be kept low and the onion simmered gently without browning or scorching until quite soft. If onion is to be *sautéed* (or fried), heat should be higher and onion should be stir-fried until evenly browned (but not burned). The flavor produced by the two methods is quite different.

Boiled Onions. Usually the small white onions are used, but large yellow ones may also be boiled; cook covered in ample boiling salted water until fork-tender. Serve 3 small onions or 1 large one to each person.

Creamed Onions. Boil onions, drain thoroughly, make a sauce by blending condensed cream of celery soup with enough milk for desired consistency.

Escalloped Onions. Prepare small whole creamed onions, place in shallow baking dish, cover with blanket of finely crushed Shredded Wheat or crushed whole-bran cereal mixed with butter and grated cheese. Bake until crumbs are nicely browned.

Stuffed Onions. Boil large onions until tender; drain and cool. Scoop out top; fill with crumbled soft whole-wheat crumbs sautéed in butter until crisp. Pack onions tightly together in baking dish; bake just until crumbs are browned.

Oven-Fried Onion Rings

½ cup whole-wheat or soy flour
1 teaspoon salt
½ teaspoon baking powder
1 egg, separated
⅓ cup milk

2 tablespoons oil
1 large Spanish onion, cut in ¼-inch slices
3 cups Wheat Chex crushed to 1 cup

Combine flour, salt, and baking powder. Beat egg white until stiff; separately beat egg yolk with milk and oil. Blend dry ingredients into yolk-milk mixture, then fold in whites. Separate onion into rings, dip each ring in batter; drain well. Dip in crumbs on both sides. Chill. Arrange on well-greased or Teflon-coated baking sheet, bake in preheated 425° F. oven, turning once, until well browned.

Parsnips. This wintertime vegetable is very high in fiber and has a natural sweetness; it is good alone and in stews. Pare with carrot scraper, cut in lengthwise halves or quarters, cook about 6 minutes in boiling salted water, then sauté briefly in butter. Serve sprinkled with parsley.

Potatoes (*White*). For those concerned about weight control the three best ways to prepare potatoes are: baked in jackets, boiled in jackets, and Parsley Potatoes. Even if skins are removed after cooking, fiber is retained, but the skins are the best fiber and mineral source. Before baking, brush outside lightly with oil, and cut a tiny hole at the end (to prevent an explosion of starch).

Parsley Potatoes. Boil thin-skinned red potatoes, without peeling, then cut in quarters, add chopped parsley and 1 teaspoon of butter.

Red Cabbage. Unless acid is added during cooking, red cabbage turns a dreary purple-gray, but if vinegar or lemon juice is added, some sweetening is necessary.

Red Cabbage with Apples

1 tablespoon butter	½ cup chopped pitted prunes
1 small onion, sliced	or raisins
1 apple, cored, sliced	Pinch of cloves
4 cups shredded red cabbage	Salt to taste
2 tablespoons vinegar or lemon juice	

Melt butter in large heavy saucepan, add onion and apple and sauté until lightly browned. Add cabbage, vinegar or lemon juice, prunes, and cloves. Cover pan, cook over low heat, stirring occasionally, until cabbage is tender (about 10 minutes). Drain off excess liquid, if any. Makes 6 servings.

With Soy Sauce. Cook 1 medium onion, sliced, in butter or oil until soft; add cabbage, 1 or 2 tablespoons of sunflower kernels *or* caraway seeds, and salt. Cover, cook without added water over low heat, stirring occasionally, for 5 minutes. Add juice of ½ lemon and 1 tablespoon of soy sauce, and continue cooking a few minutes longer if necessary. Serve topped with yogurt.

Rutabaga. Cut away heavy rind, cube the yellow "Swedish turnip," cook in salted water, covered, until fork-tender. Mash, beat in a tablespoon or so of butter, season generously with black pepper.

Snow Peas. Trim only the ends, stir-fry in oil, uncovered, or cook in boiling salted water until barely tender. They should be almost crunchy. Good combined with mushrooms and bok choy or cauliflower leaves.

Spinach. Fresh loose spinach has more flavor and food value than the plastic bags of prewashed spinach which may have been lying in the supermarket bins for a long time. Fill the sink with cold water, dump in the spinach, add a few ice cubes, and let stand for 15–20 minutes; then shake each cluster of leaves thoroughly and break leaves from stems. Prepared this way, no water need be added to the kettle; enough is retained on the leaves. Sprinkle with salt, cover tightly, and as soon as spinach is steaming, turn heat very low, cook 3–5 minutes until quite wilted, then drain thoroughly and chop as you drain. A few drops of lemon juice and a pat of butter are seasoning enough. For more fiber, stir in a few chopped sunflower kernels.

Spinach Catalan

2 pounds fresh spinach, washed
½ teaspoon salt
1 tablespoon minced onion
1 tablespoon pine nuts or chopped sunflower kernels
2 tablespoons oil
2 tablespoons dried currants, softened
Vinegar and oil, passed in cruets

Cook spinach as described above; drain and chop. In frying pan, sauté onion and nuts in oil until lightly browned. Soften currants by soaking briefly in hot water, then drain. Add onion, nuts, and currants to cooked spinach; distribute evenly. Serve warm, passing vinegar and oil. Makes 6–8 servings.

(Frozen chopped spinach, cooked first, can be used in above recipe, as can frozen collards or turnip greens, or fresh collards, or chard.)

Frozen Chopped Spinach in Wine. Only partially thaw chopped spinach, put in heavy pan with ¼ cup of red wine; sprinkle with salt and nutmeg. Cook over moderate heat, stirring, until broken up; then cover and cook for 1 minute longer. Caraway or fennel seeds may also be added.

Squash (hard rind). Winter squash, including hubbard, acorn, and butternut, is an excellent fiber source. Cut squash in half with long sturdy knife. Scoop out seeds, pulp, and string. Place in baking pan, hollow side up, with dab of butter and 1 teaspoon of honey or maple syrup; sprinkle with salt. Bake until fork-tender (45 minutes to 1½ hours, depending on size of squash). The acorn squash can be served right in the shell, one half to each person; the larger squash should be scooped out, mashed, and served from a serving dish. Season with pumpkin pie spices if desired.

Summer Squash. The thin-skinned yellow crook-neck, zucchini, and pattypan squash need not be pared, or only very lightly peeled. Cut in thick slices, cook in butter or oil (no liquid needed, they have enough of their own) with herbs.

Pattypan may be scooped out, parboiled, and used like a shell to hold a seasoned crumbed mixture (see Stuffed Onions).

Zucchini may be scrubbed with vegetable brush, scooped out to be stuffed, or sliced crosswise. Sauté in olive or sesame oil or butter with herbs such as oregano and thyme; or steam on rack over boiling water for 3 to 4 minutes.

Sweet Potatoes and Yams. For best fiber, bake these in their skins, like Idaho potatoes; serve with butter. They rank with lima beans as among the highest in calories of all vegetables but are an excellent source of Vitamin A, and one *large* yam or sweet potato contains over a gram of fiber.

Sugarless Candied Sweets

6 medium-to-large sweet potatoes or yams
6 pitted prunes, cut in halves, or 10 dates, cut in pieces
¼ cup unsweetened shredded coconut

Salt, nutmeg
Butter or margarine
½ cup orange juice

Cook potatoes in their jackets; when cool, peel off skin and cut lengthwise into slices. Place in greased casserole in layers with the fruit and coconut, sprinkling the potatoes with salt and nutmeg, and dotting with butter or margarine. Add orange juice. Bake, covered, in moderate oven (350° F.) for 30 minutes; uncover during last 10 minutes. Makes 6–8 servings.

Tomatoes. Most of what little fiber tomatoes possess is in their skins, the rest in the seeds. However, they are such an excellent source of Vitamin C that they should be served frequently, either fresh or canned. The following recipes suggest several ways in which fiber can be added to tomatoes.

Fried Tomatoes. Cut large firm unpeeled tomatoes in ¼-inch slices and dredge with a mixture of whole-wheat or soy flour and salt. Sauté in 2 or 3 tablespoons of shortening until well browned on each side, turning once. This can be done with either green or ripe tomatoes. A "gravy" can be made with those that break up when turned over: stir the tomato pulp to mash it, add a little more flour, then slowly stir in milk and cook until thickened. Serve sauce over the tomatoes.

Escalloped Tomatoes. Canned tomatoes are best for this. Place tomatoes in a baking dish, break them up with fork into pieces, sprinkle with salt and pepper and push down into the tomato liquid pieces of whole-wheat bread, about as much as the tomatoes will take. Bake uncovered until top is well browned; the liquid in the tomatoes will evaporate considerably as they bake.

Baked Stuffed Tomatoes

8 medium or 6 large
  tomatoes
Salt
4 tablespoons olive oil
1 cup chopped onion
2½ cups *cooked* millet,
  bulgur, or kasha
1 tablespoon toasted
  soybeans
2 tablespoons currants or
  raisins

1 tablespoon chopped fresh
  dill, or 1 teaspoon dried
  dillweed
¼ teaspoon black pepper
  (or to taste)
½ cup fine dry crumbs or
  finely crushed Shredded
  Wheat

Scoop out tomatoes, leaving quarter-inch shells. Reserve 1 cup of the drained pulp. Sprinkle salt over the inside of each, and brush inside and out with oil. Simmer onions in 2 tablespoons of oil until soft; add to the cooked cereal with soybeans, currants (or raisins), chopped dill, and pepper. Stir in reserved tomato pulp. Pile mixture inside the tomatoes. Over top of each spread crumbs or crushed cereal sautéed in oil. Bake in moderate oven (350° F.) for about 45 minutes. Good both hot and cold. Makes 6–8 servings.

Mixed Vegetables Estofada

2 garlic cloves
¼ cup minced ham
  (optional)
1 pimiento or red sweet
  pepper, diced
1 medium onion, chopped
3 or 4 tablespoons olive oil

2 carrots, scraped and
  quartered
1 pound green or wax beans,
  "frenched"
½ cup water
½ teaspoon salt
1 tablespoon minced parsley

Cook garlic, ham, pimiento, and onion in olive oil over low heat until onion is soft. Add carrots, beans, water, and salt; cover, cook over low heat until vegetables are tender. *Do not drain.* Serve topped with parsley. Good either hot or cold. Makes about 8 servings.

Variations: Instead of beans, add 1 10-ounce package of

artichoke hearts, or 1 cup of shelled fresh peas (or a 10-ounce package of frozen peas), or fresh or frozen lima beans, or frozen black-eyed peas.

Instead of water, add ½ cup of tomato juice, and omit ham.

OTHER SIDE DISHES

Cereals

Normally we think of the "starch foods" to be served with a meal as limited to white potatoes, rice, or pasta (spaghetti or macaroni). But millet, bulgur, and kasha all can be served as part of the meal and each is an excellent source of fiber and good nutrition.

Pastas made with white flour are the least nutritious—the lowest in fiber, the highest in calories. Whole-wheat pastas, available at health stores, offer more food value (better protein, better fiber, more vitamins and minerals). When cooked in a casserole with a sauce, these can be quite delicious. I must confess it took me a long time to get up courage to try them, though, because they look so repulsive. When at last I had bought and cooked a token amount, I felt much like English poet Matthew Arnold after his first taste of buckwheat pancakes. Arnold, while on an American tour, was entertained at the home of a Boston matron who thought he might enjoy tasting a unique American breakfast treat. After gingerly trying a snippet of ash-gray buckwheat pancake, Arnold turned to his wife to say, "Do try them, my deah. They are not hawlf as nawsty as they look."

Cooked Millet
(Basic Recipe)

1 cup millet grains	3 cups water (or seasoned
1 teaspoon salt	broth)

Place ingredients in saucepan with fitted cover, bring to a boil, lower heat, simmer gently for 20 minutes, or until all liquid is absorbed. Serve as a substitute for rice. Makes 3 cups or 4 average servings. (For 2 or 3 servings, divide ingredients by half.)

Green Millet

3 cups *cooked* millet
2 tablespoons oil
1 small-to-medium onion, chopped

Salt to taste
1 cup chopped fresh parsley
¼ cup grated cheese (optional)

Cook millet as directed in basic recipe. Sauté onion in oil until lightly browned; sprinkle with salt. Add parsley, cook for 30 seconds, then add millet and cheese and stir to blend. Keep warm in covered casserole or over hot water. Makes 4–6 servings.

Millet Pilaf

2 cups millet grains
2 tablespoons butter
½ cup blanched slivered almonds or sunflower kernels
½ cup currants or raisins
2 onions, chopped
½ teaspoon cinnamon

¼ teaspoon powdered cloves
¼ teaspoon crushed cardamom
¼ teaspoon black pepper
6 cups water
2½ teaspoons salt
3 hard-cooked eggs

Add cold water to millet grains, let stand 30 minutes, then drain. Melt butter in large heavy pot, add almonds, stir-fry until lightly browned; add currants and onions, stir-fry until onions are yellowed and soft—but do not allow to brown. Add spices and blend well. Add the drained millet, stir to glaze, then add water and salt. Bring to a boil, cover, turn heat as low as possible, and cook for 20 minutes, or until all liquid is absorbed (with tunnels through the millet grains). Uncover, place a cloth or absorbent paper over the top of the pan and keep over lowest heat for 5 minutes longer. Or transfer to a casserole and keep uncovered in warming oven until time to serve. Place slices of hard-cooked egg over top. Makes 10 servings. Excellent with roast chicken, or as an entree in a vegetarian meal.

Simple Bulgur Pilaf

1 medium onion, chopped	1–1½ teaspoons salt
2 tablespoons oil	1 tablespoon sunflower
1 cup bulgur	kernels, pine nuts, or
2 cups water or broth	raisins (optional)

Sauté onion in oil until lightly browned; add bulgur, stir to coat with oil; add water or seasoned broth and salt (use less salt if using broth). Stir in nuts or fruit if desired. Bring to a boil, cover, reduce heat, cook at low heat until all liquid is absorbed (20–30 minutes). Let stand for 5 minutes. Serve hot. Makes 4–5 servings.

Kasha

2 tablespoons margarine	2½ cups boiling water or
1 small-to-medium onion,	broth
chopped	1 egg, beaten (optional)
¼–½ teaspoon salt	¼ cup chopped parsley
1 cup Wolff's kasha	
(cracked buckwheat)	

Melt margarine, add onion, and cook, stirring, until lightly browned. Add salt and kasha; stir to blend. (Some instructions suggest adding a beaten egg to the kasha grains first, then heating this mixture, stirring constantly, in an ungreased skillet. I tried this but found no advantage in it—the grains remain chewy when water is added directly to them.) Add *boiling* water, stirring in slowly, then bring water again to the boil. Cover, lower heat, cook until all liquid is absorbed and grains are tender. If desired, stir in a beaten egg quickly, as for fried rice, then stir in parsley. (But both these additions are optional.) Makes 4–6 servings.

Brown Rice

To shorten cooking time, about ½–1 hour before cooking, place rice in a saucepan; for each cup of rice, add 2½ cups of *boiling* water and 1 teaspoon of salt. Cover, let stand. When ready to cook, reheat, using the same water, until it reaches a boil. Lower heat, cook 30–35 minutes until all liquid is absorbed. Rice will be fluffier if placed uncovered in a warming oven for another 10–15 minutes. One cup of rice becomes 3 cups after cooking, which makes 4–6 servings.

Mixed Cereal Grains

For a vegetarian meal, a mixture of cereal grains cooked together is interesting. First heat 3 cups of water and ½ teaspoon of salt to boiling point, add a total of 1 cup cereal: millet and bulgur make an excellent combination, or combine buckwheat grains, rye, or triticale flakes with brown rice. Cook covered for about ½ hour, then let stand overnight and reheat, covered, in the oven for about ½ hour. To speed cooking, put all the grains through the food grinder; keep stored in jars to use as needed.

Oven-Baked Rice

Either white or brown rice may be cooked this way and it's more foolproof than top-of-stove. Place rice, salt, and 1 tablespoon of butter in a casserole. Add *boiling* water—the same proportion as in top-of-stove recipes. (Normally 2 cups of water to 1 cup of converted long-grain white rice, and 2¼–2½ cups of water to 1 cup of brown rice.) Cover tightly, bake for a total of 40–55 minutes in a moderate oven until all liquid is absorbed. Stir once after first half hour. If it remains in oven longer than this, rice should remain moist as long as it is tightly covered.

Yellow Rice with Pigeon Peas

This is a Caribbean favorite. The pigeon peas, *gandules,* are native to the Caribbean but usually will be found in Latin American groceries, both fresh and canned. Gandules are higher in fiber than our green peas.

1 can (1 pound) gandules
½ cup chopped onion
2 tablespoons fat or oil
Pinch of achiote powder
1 or 2 garlic cloves, minced
1 green pepper, seeded and minced

1 light green or red sweet chili pepper, minced
½ teaspoon oregano
½ tablespoon salt
1½ cups converted long-grain rice
3 cups liquid

Drain canned peas, saving liquid. (If fresh peas are used, cook separately in advance.) Cook onion in fat or oil, adding achiote powder; add garlic, the two kinds of peppers, and oregano. Cook until soft. Add peas, uncooked rice, salt, and reserved liquid plus water to make 3 cups. Cover, bring to a boil, reduce heat, and cook until liquid is absorbed (about 20 minutes). Makes 6 servings. (Brown rice is not suitable for this dish.)

Pilaf Variations

(Use millet, rice or bulgur.)

• First sauté green or red sweet pepper with onion, then add rice or other cereal grains.

• Use tomato juice or canned tomatoes for part or all of liquid.

• Add diced carrots with rice or other cereal; cook for same length of time.

• Mexican style: add kernel corn (scraped from cob or canned), sliced or chopped pitted black olives, taste of onion.

• Add almost any nuts or seeds: chopped peanuts, sunflower kernels, caraway seeds, cumin seeds, slivered toasted almonds, chopped walnuts.

Dried Legumes

In the big family of legumes, all these are members: yellow and green split peas, black-eyed peas, chickpeas (garbanzos), gandules (pigeon peas), the tiny red or pink lentils and the larger brown or green lentils, soybeans, mung beans, limas, kidney beans, pinto and black beans, and several varieties of white beans, also fava beans. Most need presoaking or very long cooking, or both. If not cooked sufficiently, they are hard to digest and cause flatulence.

Neither split peas nor lentils need presoaking, however, and the tiny little red (or pink) lentils cook almost as quickly as rice. (And they are bland enough to be served in place of rice with certain stews or curries.)

Many people swear by pressure cookers for dried legumes: it requires only 45 minutes from start to finish at 15 pounds pressure. But the petcock can become clogged, a mess to clean up. The electric crock-pot is better in many ways; no matter how many hours of cooking are required, no watching is needed, and long cooking brings out flavor.

To shorten top-of-stove cooking, soak beans by covering with *boiling water* (no salt), bring water again to boil, turn off heat. Let stand for an hour or overnight, whichever is best for your schedule, then bring slowly again to boil (do not drain), add more liquid as needed, simmer gently, tightly covered, until tender. When dried beans seem to take forever to become tender, it is because of overlong shelf age.

For a household of four or more, it pays to buy dried legumes in bulk—they cost less than a fourth as much. But for small households, or those households that have only two adult eaters, the canned beans or peas may be worth the extra cost in convenience. When a big quantity is prepared, it seems to take forever to finish it.

Curried Dahl

3 tablespoons butter or oil
1 tablespoon cumin or fennel seeds*
1 medium onion, thinly sliced
1 large garlic clove, slit
2 bay leaves, crumbled (optional)
2 tablespoons curry powder
¼ teaspoon *each*:
    nutmeg
    powdered ginger
    turmeric or dry mustard
    cayenne pepper

¼ cup chopped fresh coriander, or 1 tablespoon crushed coriander
2 fully ripe tomatoes, peeled and chopped, or 1 cup canned tomatoes
1½ cups tiny red lentils
1½ teaspoons salt
4½ cups water

To the melted butter or oil, add the cumin or fennel seeds and stir-fry until browned. Add onion and garlic, cook until soft. Press garlic into fat to release juices. Add the spices, stir-fry over low heat for 1 or 2 minutes. Add fresh or crushed coriander and tomato, cook for 2 minutes, then add lentils, salt, and water. Bring to a boil, lower heat, cover, cook until lentils are soft (about 30 minutes). Delectable with ham or pork or as part of a vegetarian meal. Makes 10–12 servings. (Divide all ingredients by half to serve 4 or 5 persons.)

*If fennel seeds are used, add ½ teaspoon of cumin powder; if cumin seeds are used, add crushed fennel.

Simple Dahl

When pink lentils are to be served as a side dish with a curry or a meat stew, this is a delicious and easy way to prepare them. Sauté onions in oil or butter until soft and lightly browned; add 1 teaspoon of salt plus any other seasonings desired. (A dash of ginger helps.) Add 1 cup of lentils, then 2 cups of water. Bring to a boil, cover, lower heat, and cook for 25–30 minutes, or until tender and water is absorbed. Makes about 3 servings.

Refried Beans

1 pound dried pinto or black beans
9 cups boiling water
2 tablespoons oil
2 teaspoons salt

2 large onions, minced or grated
¼ teaspoon cumin
3 garlic cloves, crushed

Wash beans in cold water, drain, add to rapidly boiling water in a large kettle. When water has returned to the boil, turn off heat, let stand for 1 hour, then turn on heat again, bring water again to a boil, reduce heat, and cook slowly for 1 hour. Add remaining ingredients and continue cooking until beans are very tender. Drain off excess water, leaving about ½ cup, so beans will puree easily. Mash with potato masher or beat in blender or with electric beater. Makes about 5 cups. Can be kept in refrigerator, covered, for some time, to use as needed with Mexican meals.

Lentil Pottage

3 or 4 large yellow onions
½ cup olive oil
1 cup brown lentils
6–7 cups water

1 cup long-grain converted rice
1 tablespoon salt
Minced parsley

Cut each onion in half, then in sticks. Sauté slowly, stirring frequently, in the olive oil until well browned but not scorched. (Important to the flavor of the dish is the even browning of the onions.) At the same time, cook the lentils separately in water (no salt) for 35–45 minutes. Add the onions, the rice, and salt; cook about 25 minutes longer, or until all liquid is absorbed and lentils are tender. Serve garnished with minced parsley. Surprisingly, this is as good cold as hot. In the Middle East, where it is a favorite dish, it is most frequently served lukewarm, sprinkled with lemon juice just before serving. Makes 8 servings.

Garbanzos with Yams

Cook 2 medium-sized yams in their jackets until tender; drain, peel off skins, cut in quarters or dice. Combine with 1 can (1 pound) or 2 cups of cooked, well-drained chickpeas, 2 tablespoons of chopped parsley, and ½ tablespoon of butter; mix well. Makes 4–6 servings.

Sesame Almond Noodles

3 tablespoons sesame seeds
½ cup slivered blanched
   almonds
2 tablespoons butter or oil
Dash of MSG (optional)

½ teaspoon salt
3 cups hot cooked whole-
   wheat or green noodles
   (1½ cups before cooking)
¼–½ cup chopped parsley

Stir-fry sesame seeds and almonds in butter or oil until golden; add seasonings. Add to noodles, toss to blend. Add parsley, toss again. Makes 4 servings.

Baked Stuffing with Limas

This could, I suppose, actually be used as a stuffing, but it is intended as a side dish.

2 quarts stale cubes of
   whole-wheat or other
   health bread
4 tablespoons butter or
   margarine
1 medium onion, chopped
1 teaspoon salt
¼ teaspoon pepper
½ teaspoon thyme

¼ cup chopped parsley
½ cup chopped celery
1 10-ounce package frozen
   limas, cooked
¼ cup chopped ripe olives
2 eggs, slightly beaten
1½ cups chicken or
   vegetable broth

Bread should be cut into ½-inch cubes. Melt butter, add onion and seasonings; cook until onion is soft. Add to bread with remaining ingredients, stir to blend thoroughly. Pack into well-greased 1½-quart baking dish. If dish does not have its own cover, cover with foil. Bake in moderate oven for 45 minutes. Serve with gravy, to accompany roast meat or poultry, or as part of a vegetarian dinner. Makes 6–8 servings.

CHAPTER 11

Salads from First Course to Dessert

Tossed salads are wonderful for health, an excellent source of fiber, and *can* be low in calories—depending to a large extent on the dressing used. The best of all dressings for tossed salads is the simplest: a fragrant oil (my preference is olive oil), vinegar or lemon juice, and salt—nothing else. Very little oil is required: a few tablespoons is enough for quite a large bowl of salad.

Besides high-fiber vegetables, toss into the bowl fruits, salad greens, an assortment of other fibrous goodies such as cooked bean or peas, nuts, soybeans, sunflower kernels, buckwheat grains or groats, wheat flakes or berries, whole-bran cereal, toasted croutons of whole wheat (or Wheat Chex). (Some of these are individually fairly high in calorie content, but since the quantity added is so small, the per-serving amount remains minimal.)

I feel impelled to add a footnote about the oil: A few years ago when I visited Crete, the tourist guide commented that they had virtually no cases of cancer on the island, which she attributed to their daily use of olive oil. At the time, gazing up at the unpolluted blue sky and observing their pastoral life-style, I thought, but how could people here be anything but healthy? Yet olive oil is as effective as bran in assisting with the removal of wastes, so perhaps she was on target at that!

Serving salad as a first course has several advantages. It helps to take the edge off appetite in a low-calorie way, and serving it first is one way of making sure it will be eaten. When it is served later, it could be passed up.

Tossed Salad

The fun of mixing a tossed salad is putting together unlikely combinations. Almost any of the following may be combined in any way you like.

The Greens
Bibb lettuce
leaf lettuce
Boston lettuce
romaine
curly endive
Belgian endive
escarole
watercress
raw spinach
celery cabbage

Raw Vegetables
avocado, sliced or diced
chopped celery
shredded or grated carrot
chopped scallion
thin-sliced onion
slivers of white turnip
green pepper
red sweet pepper
cherry tomatoes
sliced or quartered tomatoes
radishes, red or white
cucumber
tender green beans
raw beet greens, chopped
celery cabbage
dandelion greens
mustard greens
shredded red or green cabbage
shredded cauliflower leaves
sliced raw cauliflower
celery leaves
Italian parsley

Cooked or Canned Vegetables
artichoke hearts
asparagus spears
beets, whole or sliced
water chestnuts, sliced
bamboo shoots
potatoes, cooked
green beans

Fruits
diced oranges
sliced apples
seedless grapes
seeded black or red grapes
raisins or currants
grapefruit segments

Nuts, Seeds, Grains
cumin seeds
fennel seeds
caraway seeds
sunflower kernels
toasted soybeans
buckwheat grains
rye or wheat flakes
toasted sesame seeds

*Cooked or Canned
   Vegetables*
lima beans
red kidney beans
wax beans
green peas
chickpeas
hearts of palm
black and green
   olives
leftover cooked
   vegetables (any
   but those of the
   cabbage family)

Nuts, Seeds, Grains
whole-wheat
   croutons
Wheat Chex
wheat germ

Oil-Vinegar Dressing

Salt
3 tablespoons olive or other salad oil
1 tablespoon vinegar

First sprinkle salad ingredients with salt from a shaker, then add oil. Toss to coat all ingredients, then sprinkle with vinegar. This is enough dressing for 4–6 cups of tossed salad. Double ingredients for 8–12 cups of salad. The best time to add the dressing is at the table.

Sweet (Sugarless) Dressing

½ teaspoon salt or seasoned
   salt
2 tablespoons olive oil
2 scallions, minced, or 4
   or 5 very thin slices of
   onion

1 tablespoon vinegar or
   lemon juice
1 orange, peeled, cut in
   chunks, or
1 tablespoon orange juice
   (fresh, not frozen)

Combine all ingredients in salad bowl at least an hour before serving. The onion and the orange juice together provide all the sweetening that's needed. This should be ample dressing for 4–6 cups of salad.

Yogurt Salad Dressing

½ teaspoon salt or seasoned
  salt
1 garlic clove, crushed
2 or 3 scallions, minced, or
  ¼ cup minced onion
2 tablespoons chopped
  parsley

2 tablespoons oil
¼–½ cup plain yogurt
  (to taste)
½ teaspoon grated lemon
  rind

Combine ingredients in order given, beating to blend completely. Prepare ahead; chill. Beat again just before serving. Makes ⅓–⅔ cup of dressing.

Yogurt Roquefort Dressing

¼ cup crumbled blue cheese
½ cup plain yogurt
Salt to taste

½ teaspoon dry or Dijon
  mustard

Combine ingredients; beat until fairly smooth. Makes ¾ cup of dressing.

Vinaigrette Dressing

1 garlic clove
½ teaspoon salt
½ teaspoon dry or prepared
  mustard
2 tablespoons capers, drained
½ teaspoon grated lemon
  rind
2 tablespoons minced green
  pepper

2 or 3 scallions, minced, or
  1 tablespoon grated onion
1 hard-cooked egg, minced
3 tablespoons oil
1 tablespoon vinegar or
  lemon juice, or ½ tablespoon of each

Crush garlic in bowl in which dressing is to be mixed, using a wooden pestle. When crushed to shreds, the shreds may be removed (the juice and flavor will remain). Add remaining ingredients; marinate ½–1 hour before adding to salad. (A teaspoon of instant minced onion may be used instead of the scallion or grated onion.) Makes about ⅓ cup.

Yogurt Horseradish Dressing

This is best for solid ingredients, not suitable for greens.

1 teaspoon grated horse-
  radish
½ cup plain yogurt
Freshly ground black pepper

Pinch of dry mustard or
  ginger
Grated onion to taste

Combine all ingredients. Makes ½ cup.

Orange and Avocado Salad

(LC)

2 seedless oranges
1 small onion, thinly sliced
1 ripe avocado, sliced
2 tablespoons lemon juice
2 tablespoons vinegar
½ cup olive oil

Pinch of curry powder
  (optional)
Salt, pepper
8–10 pimiento-stuffed olives,
  sliced
4–6 cups mixed greens

Peel oranges so no white remains on outside; dice right
through segments. Place in salad bowl with onion and avocado; add lemon juice, stirring so avocado is completely covered.
Add vinegar, oil, curry powder, salt, and pepper. Cover
tightly with plastic wrap; marinate for 1 hour. Add olives and
greens just before serving. Makes 8 servings.

Egg and Bean Salad

(LC)

1 cup cooked or canned
  green beans
1 cup cooked lima beans
½ cup cooked or canned red
  kidney beans
Few slices onion

2 tablespoons olive oil
2 tablespoons lemon juice or
  vinegar
Salt, pepper
4–6 cups mixed salad greens
3 hard-cooked eggs, sliced

Place all beans in bowl with onion, olive oil, lemon juice or
vinegar; add seasonings, marinate for 1 hour. Add salad
greens; toss. Serve with egg slices over top, to be tossed at
table. Makes about 8 servings.

Canadian Apple Salad

(LC)

2 cups diced red Delicious or Winesap apples, not peeled
1 tablespoon lemon juice
½ cup diced celery
¼ cup chopped walnuts (optional)

1 tablespoon olive oil
Salt, pepper
Salad greens
Yogurt Roquefort Dressing

Place apples in salad bowl, sprinkle with lemon juice, toss to moisten apples with the juice. Add celery, walnuts, oil, and seasonings. Marinate, covered, until time to serve, then add salad greens and dressing. Makes 4–6 servings.

Winter Salad

2 large tart red apples, seeded, chopped, not peeled
1 celery stalk, minced
6 walnuts or pecans, chopped
2 raw white turnips, cut in sticks

½ green pepper, chopped
8 pitted dates, chopped
Pinch of curry powder
¼ cup Oil-Vinegar Dressing
Mixed salad greens

Combine all ingredients but salad greens; toss to blend, marinate until needed, then add to salad greens. Makes 6–8 servings. (To make this qualify as a low-calorie salad, use 1 tablespoon of sunflower kernels instead of nuts; omit dates.)

Coleslaw
(Basic Recipe)

(LC)

2 cups shredded white or green cabbage
1 teaspoon salt
¼ teaspoon dry mustard
1–1½ tablespoons vinegar or lemon juice

1 tablespoon olive oil
1½ tablespoons sour cream or plain yogurt

Place shredded cabbage in bowl, add salt and mustard, stir to coat. Add vinegar or lemon juice and oil; toss. Add one or more additional ingredients as suggested in the following variations, along with the sour cream or yogurt; blend well. Makes 4–6 servings. (If a creamier slaw is preferred, add 1 tablespoon of mayonnaise—but no more.)

Apple Coleslaw

Add 1 red apple, cored, chopped, and ¼ cup of chopped peanuts.

Carrot Coleslaw

Add 1 carrot, coarsely grated, 1 tablespoon of chopped parsley, and a dash of cayenne or paprika.

Pineapple Coleslaw

Add 1 cup of well-drained crushed pineapple, ½ cup of minced green pepper, and 1 tablespoon of minced fresh or frozen dill.

Nutty Coleslaw

Add ¼ cup of sunflower kernels and ¼ cup of toasted soybeans or peanuts, chopped.

Seeded Coleslaw

Add 1 teaspoon of poppy seeds, toasted sesame seeds, caraway or fennel seeds.

Red Cabbage Slaw I

(LC)

4 cups finely shredded red cabbage, chopped
¼–½ cup chopped green pepper
1 white turnip, in sticks, or ½ cup sliced white radishes
1 tablespoon toasted sunflower kernels

1 teaspoon caraway seeds
4 or 5 thin slices onion
½ teaspoon seasoned salt
Dash of ginger, black pepper
3 tablespoons olive oil
½ tablespoon lemon juice

Combine first five ingredients in salad bowl. Combine remaining ingredients separately to make the dressing; marinate for ½ hour or longer. Add to cabbage mixture just before serving. Makes 6–8 servings.

Red Cabbage Slaw II

(LC)

2 cups chopped red cabbage
¼–½ cup sliced raw mushrooms
1 apple, cored, sliced (not peeled)
½ green pepper, chopped

1–2 tablespoons toasted soybeans
Salt to taste
2 tablespoons olive oil
½ tablespoon vinegar
Shredded mixed salad greens

Combine all ingredients but salad greens; blend well. Add salad greens just before serving. Makes 3 or 4 servings.

Apple Spinach Salad

(LC)

1 tart firm apple
2 tablespoons lemon juice
3–4 tablespoons olive oil
2 scallions, minced
1 teaspoon dried mint, crumbled
½ teaspoon salt

⅛ teaspoon curry powder
1 tablespoon capers
1 pound fresh spinach (not packaged)
6 or 8 radishes, sliced
2 tablespoons sunflower kernels

Quarter apple, cut out seeds, then thinly slice. Place in small bowl and sprinkle with lemon juice, toss, then add oil, scallion, mint, and other seasonings, and the capers. Marinate until time to serve. Place spinach in sink, add water to cover and a few ice cubes, let stand in water for 5 minutes, then shake to rid leaves of both grit and excess water. Remove stems; cut larger leaves in small pieces. Chill in large plastic bag until time to serve. Then place in salad bowl with marinated apple mixture and remaining ingredients; toss to blend. Makes about 6 servings.

Spinach Orange Salad

Use 1 medium navel orange, peeled and diced, instead of the apple in the above recipe.

Mimosa Salad

(LC)

2 or 3 scallions, minced
2 tablespoons chopped green pepper
½ cup Oil-Vinegar Dressing
Seasoned salt

Other condiments to taste
3 hard-cooked eggs
1 pound fresh leaf spinach
½ cup bacon-flavored vegetable protein bits

Combine scallion, green pepper, dressing, and other seasonings to taste. Separate yolks from whites of hard-cooked eggs. Mince the whites, add to dressing. Sieve yolks, set aside.

Prepare spinach as described in preceding recipe. Chill until time to serve. Then place spinach in salad bowl, add bacon-flavored bits and dressing; toss to blend. Sprinkle sieved egg yolk over top and, at table, toss once more. Makes about 6 servings.

Salade Algerienne

4 anchovy fillets, chopped
2 hard-cooked egg yolks
2 tablespoons minced parsley
1 teaspoon cumin seeds
3 tablespoons olive oil
1 tablespoon lemon juice or vinegar
Salt, pepper to taste
Several sprigs of fresh basil, minced

4 green peppers, seeded and diced
1 small onion, thinly sliced
½ cup thinly sliced cucumber
4–6 fully ripe tomatoes, chopped or quartered
1 cup black olives
Lettuce

Crush anchovy fillets with yolks of eggs, parsley, and cumin seeds; work in oil to form a paste. Add lemon juice, taste for salt—it may not need any more than the anchovies supply. Add pepper and basil, pour over mixture of green peppers, onion, and cucumber. Marinate until time to serve, then combine with tomatoes, olives, and lettuce. Makes 8–10 servings.

Greek Salad with Feta Cheese

The ingredients for this salad vary according to what's on the market. But always included are tomatoes, green pepper, lettuce, black olives, and feta cheese. Sometimes cooked dried beans are added, sometimes artichoke hearts, cucumbers, or onions. The dressing is always simply salt, olive oil, and lemon juice, added when the salad is served.

Celeriac Salad

2 cups celeriac, cut in
  julienne sticks
1 cup carrots, julienned or
  coarsely grated
¼ teaspoon celery seeds
1 teaspoon toasted sesame
  seeds

Salt, pepper to taste
2 tablespoons olive oil
1 tablespoon lemon juice
2 tablespoons sweet or sour
  cream

Combine ingredients in order given, but add the cream just before serving. This is most frequently served as part of an hors d'oeuvres variées. Makes 3 cups, about 6–8 hors d'oeuvres servings.

Springtime Salad

(LC)

2 cups fresh young dandelion
  leaves, torn in pieces
1 cup shredded wild mustard
  leaves
1 cup watercress, stems
  partially removed

2 cups fresh spinach leaves
6 or 8 radishes, sliced
½ cup Oil-Vinegar Dressing

Everyone knows what dandelion leaves look like—but be sure to dig up the plants when they are still young and not yet bitter. Mustard greens are usually to be found in the woods, or may grow along the roadside. In the woods, also, are to be found fiddleheads, which look like tiny ferns about to bud. If you haven't time to go looking for them, perhaps there will be some leaves culled from plants in the garden that needed thinning out. Combine greens and radishes, wash well, shake off excess water, and chill in plastic bag until very crisp. Toss with dressing at table. Makes 8–12 servings.

Turnip Salad

(LC)

½ cup plain yogurt or sour cream
1 tablespoon cider vinegar
2 tablespoons minced fresh onion
2 tablespoons minced parsley

1 teaspoon brown sugar
1 teaspoon salt
Dash of pepper
4 cups shredded white turnip
1 crisp apple, cored and diced (not peeled)

Combine yogurt or sour cream, vinegar, onion, parsley, sugar, salt, and pepper. Add turnip and apple; mix well. Chill for several hours. Sprinkle with additional minced parsley before serving. Serves 6–8.

Luncheon or Buffet Salads

Most of the following are filling enough to serve as a main course at lunch, or as part of a buffet spread. For hors d'oeuvres salads, see Chapter 2.

Rhinelander Herring Salad

(LC)

1 jar pickled herring, drained
½ cup diced cooked beets, drained
½ cup chopped red apple, not peeled
2 medium potatoes, cooked and diced
1 small white or yellow onion, minced
½ cup chopped walnuts or sunflower "nuts"

1 teaspoon celery seeds
¼ cup sour cream
2 tablespoons mayonnaise
1 teaspoon Dijon mustard
Sliced hard-cooked egg for garnish
2 tablespoons chopped parsley
Small whole beets (optional)

Combine herring with beets, apple, potatoes, onion, nuts, and celery seed. Blend together sour cream, mayonnaise, and mustard; add to salad mixture with parsley. Season to taste. Form into a mound and arrange sliced egg over the top. Small whole beets may be placed around the sides as well. Makes 8–10 hors d'oeuvres servings.

Salade Niçoise

3 medium potatoes, cooked in jackets
¼ cup chopped scallion
Oil-Vinegar Dressing
½ pound cooked frenched green beans
¼ cup chopped celery or celery root

½ cup Greek black olives
¼ cup sunflower kernels
1 tablespoon capers
1 6-ounce can tuna, drained
Lettuce
2 hard-cooked eggs, quartered
Pimiento strips

Peel potatoes, chop in small pieces. Add chopped scallion and part of the Oil-Vinegar Dressing. Add cooked beans, celery, black olives, sunflower kernels, and capers. Moisten with additional dressing. Then add tuna, mixing lightly so as not to break it up. Arrange salad over lettuce, garnish with additional black olives, quartered eggs, and strips of pimiento. Makes enough to serve about 8 persons as an hors d'oeuvres, 4–6 as a luncheon salad.

Luncheon Meat Salad

1 cup chopped cooked meat: roast beef, ham, salami, corned beef
1 cup cooked green peas or green beans
1 garlic clove, crushed
¼ cup chopped celery
¼ cup chopped green pepper

2 tablespoons toasted soy-beans
1 tablespoon chopped parsley
1–2 tablespoons oil
½–1 tablespoon vinegar
1–2 tablespoons mayonnaise
Salt, pepper, other seasonings to taste

Combine all ingredients; blend well. Chill. Makes about 2½ cups, or 4 servings for a luncheon salad.

Garbanzo Salad

2 cups cooked or canned
  chickpeas
3 scallions, chopped
1 or 2 garlic cloves, crushed
1 large tomato, chopped
¼ cup chopped sweet red
  peppers

¼ cup minced parsley
2 tablespoons vinegar
½ teaspoon salt
Freshly ground black pepper

Combine all ingredients, blend well; marinate several hours
before serving. Makes 8 hors d'oeuvres or 4 luncheon servings.

Greek Bean Salad

Like Garbanzo Salad but use cooked dried white beans instead
of garbanzos, green pepper instead of sweet red pepper.

Gelatin Salads

Few gelatin salads can qualify for the high-fiber diet because
they include sugar. The so-called fruit-flavored gelatins are as
much as 85 percent sugar, about 14 percent gelatin, the rest
chemicals and artificial colors and flavors. None contain *natural* fruit flavor. The only difference between gelatins labeled
"lemon-flavored" and "cherry-flavored," for example, is in
the *artificial* color and flavor added to the mixture.

Most of the recipes calling for unflavored gelatin, a pure
protein derivative, also include sugar in the ingredient list, but
in the four that follow here, I have managed to omit sugar
entirely, and there's no need for additional sweetening.

Stuffed Tomatoes in Aspic

(LC)

8 large tomatoes
1 cup diced cooked chicken
½ cup sunflower kernels
½ cup chopped green pepper
½ teaspoon celery seed
Salt, pepper, cumin to taste
16 pimiento-stuffed olives

1 envelope unflavored
  gelatin
¼ cup cold water
1½ cups clear chicken broth
2 hard-cooked eggs, sliced
Watercress

Scoop out centers of tomatoes, leaving a quarter-inch shell. Chop up tomato pulp, mix with chicken, sunflower kernels, green pepper, celery seed, and seasonings. Add 8 of the olives, chopped.

Soften gelatin in cold water; add broth heated to boiling, stir until dissolved.

Sprinkle inside of tomatoes with salt, spoon into each about 1 teaspoon of the liquid gelatin. Fill tomatoes with chicken mixture until almost but not quite to top. Spoon more gelatin over mixture, then add more stuffing to fill completely.

Place tomatoes on rack over baking sheet; spoon gelatin over outside of tomatoes as well as over stuffing. Chill until partially set. Place a slice of egg over each tomato; glaze with gelatin. Add slices of stuffed olive around the egg and spoon over more gelatin. Chill until completely set. Serve tomatoes over a bed of watercress. Pass Yogurt Bran Dressing. Makes 8 servings.

Yogurt Bran Dressing

Combine ¼ cup of plain yogurt, ¼ cup of mayonnaise, 1 teaspoon of grated horseradish, ½ teaspoon of Dijon mustard, and 1 tablespoon of whole-bran cereal. Makes ½ cup.

Tunafish Salad Mold

(LC)

1 envelope unflavored gelatin
½ cup cold water
2 egg yolks
1¼ cups skim milk
1 teaspoon salt
Dash of pepper
1 can (6 or 7 ounces) tuna, drained
½ teaspoon dry mustard
1 tablespoon lemon juice
½ cup chopped celery
½ cup chopped green pepper
½ cup grated carrot
2 tablespoons chopped sunflower or pumpkin seeds (optional)
Salad greens

Sprinkle gelatin over cold water to soften. Beat together egg yolks and milk, add salt and pepper; cook over very low heat, stirring constantly, until thickened (about 8 minutes). Remove from heat; add softened gelatin, stir until dissolved.

Place in refrigerator until it thickens to unbeaten egg-white consistency. Meantime, combine tuna with mustard, lemon juice, celery, green pepper, carrot, and seeds (put through grinder or chopped very fine). Fold into gelatin mixture, spoon into a 4-cup mold or 1-quart ring mold, or 6 individual ¾-cup molds. Chill until firm. Unmold on salad greens. Serve with Yogurt Horseradish Dressing. Makes 6 luncheon servings.

Golden Glow Salad

(LC)

1 envelope unflavored gelatin
½ teaspoon salt
1¼ cups water
⅓ cup juice drained from canned pineapple

1 teaspoon lemon juice
¾ cup well-drained crushed pineapple
¼ cup finely chopped celery
1 cup grated raw carrot
Watercress

Place gelatin, salt, and water in a saucepan, stir over low heat constantly until gelatin is dissolved. Remove from heat; add pineapple juice and lemon juice. Chill until thickened to consistency of unbeaten egg white. Fold in crushed pineapple, celery, and carrots. Pour into an 8x8-inch pan. Chill until very firm (about 3 hours). Unmold. Cut into squares. Serve on watercress with Yogurt Roquefort Dressing. Makes 6–8 servings.

Pickled Beet Ring

(LC)

1 envelope unflavored gelatin
½ cup cold water
1 cup beet juice
2 tablespoons vinegar
1 tablespoon horseradish
½ teaspoon salt
2 tablespoons grated onion
1-pound can pickled beets, drained
½ cup diced celery

½ cup diced unpeeled red apple
Salad greens
1 cup creamed cottage cheese
2 tablespoons toasted soybeans
2 tablespoons minced green pepper

Soften gelatin in cold water. Heat beet juice (drained from can of beets, with water to make 1 cup) until very hot; add to gelatin, stir until dissolved. Add vinegar, horseradish, salt, and onion. Cool until syrupy. Chop drained beets; add with celery and apple to gelatin mixture, stirring to distribute evenly. Pour into a 1-quart ring mold. Chill until very firm. Unmold on salad greens. To cottage cheese, add soybeans and green pepper, blend well; spoon mixture into center of ring mold. Makes 6–8 servings.

Fruit Salads

All of the following are suitable for serving either as a first-course fruit cup or as a dessert salad.

Orange-Blackberry-Grape Cup

When blackberries are in season, combine 1 pint of fresh berries with 1 cut-up navel orange and ½ cup of Tokay grapes (cut in halves and seeded). Add 1 tablespoon of brown sugar to the mixture; spoon into sherbet glasses. Over each sprinkle 1 teaspoon of white wine. Makes 4 or 5 servings. (When blackberries are not in season, use frozen red raspberries, well drained; sprinkle some of raspberry syrup over the fruit mixture instead of brown sugar.)

Apple Pineapple Cup

(LC)

Combine slivers of unpeeled red Delicious apple with chunks of fresh or frozen pineapple and chopped pitted dates. Add just enough Yogurt Honey Dressing to moisten.

Yogurt Honey Dressing

Combine ½ cup of plain yogurt, 1 tablespoon of wildflower or orange blossom honey, 1 teaspoon of toasted sesame seeds, and ½ teaspoon of crumbled dried tarragon. Makes ½ cup.

Blueberry Melon Salad

(LC)

For 8 servings, combine in a glass bowl 1 pint of fresh blue-berries (or thawed frozen unsweetened whole berries), 1 large pear, cored and cut in slivers, 1 cup of cantaloupe balls (or cubes), and 1 cup of honeydew melon balls (or cubes). Sweeten with apricot juice or nectar. Sprinkle shredded coconut over top.

Strawberry Nut Salad

(LC)

For 6 servings, combine in a bowl 1 pint of strawberries (washed, trimmed, cut in halves) and 2 navel oranges, diced. (Cut up oranges over the bowl so none of the juice will be lost.) Marinate the two fruits together for at least an hour before serving. The orange juice should be sweetening enough, but if you feel it must have more, sprinkle over the top 1 tablespoon of sugar. Just before serving, add ⅓ cup of coarsely chopped walnuts or pecans or shredded unsweetened coconut.

CHAPTER 12

Sandwiches, Snacks, and Drinks

The recipes in this chapter are intended primarily for children and teen-agers, though I hope adults will enjoy them, too. The sandwich fillings are suitable for school lunchboxes, or to be kept in the refrigerator for after-school snacks.

To deprive children entirely of sweets is almost impossible, since they probably will get them away from home no matter how stern you may be on the subject under your own roof. But at home certainly the snacks high in sugar and other refined carbohydrates should be kept to a minimum and desserts devised which provide important nutrients and plenty of fiber —to carry off that excess sucrose.

Nutritious drinks may be made of cocoa and chocolate, both of which are good fiber sources. Cocoa—the pure powder, not the instant mix—is higher in fiber proportionately than chocolate, because chocolate also contains fat and liquid.

But a better fiber source than either of these is carob powder, which is very similar in color and taste. Like cocoa, carob is ground from a pod, the pod of the tropical carob tree. Not only does it have more fiber proportionately, but it is considerably lower in calories; it contains only half as much fat as cocoa and has natural sweetness, so that less additional sweetening is needed.

For mothers too busy to bake cookies and whole-grain breads and crackers, there are now many good health breads available, both in health stores and at supermarkets, and nutritious snacks also exist—but they must be searched for. Sesame crackers or sticks, if made with whole-wheat or soy flour, Triscuits, Wheat Thins, yogurt chips, and *whole-wheat pretzels* are recommended.

Popcorn is no better than white bread: one cup of popcorn contains only one tenth of a gram of fiber and, with refined vegetable oil and salt added, becomes another "empty-caloried" snack. Graham crackers, long considered a health food, today are made mostly of white flour and sugar with a little "graham" (whole-wheat) flour fourth or fifth on the ingredient list.

Worst of the snack foods promoted commercially as "good for" children are the highly sugared breakfast cereals which many children munch right out of the box. Many of these also contain artificial coloring (which some pediatricians believe is a cause of the hyperactive syndrome in children).

Dried fruits make excellent snacks, as do fresh fruits. Both should always be available. Nuts, though good for fiber and high in protein, are so high in fat that when consumed nonstop, as so many children and teen-agers bolt them down, they can bring on stomach disorders besides causing acne. Excess sugar is also a cause of acne.

Raw or freshly made peanut butter is excellent, but most commercial peanut butters have added sugar or honey and the spread has been hydrogenated to increase volume. Some "peanut spreads" now on the market contain only 52 to 69 percent peanuts; the rest consists of sweeteners, fillers, and artificial flavors. Peanut butter can be made at home easily with a peanut-butter machine. It can also be made with a regular blender, although the blades tend to clog up. Many health stores sell their own fresh peanut butter with no other ingredients added.

Sandwich Fillings

Hopefully your children will accept sandwiches made with whole-wheat or other whole-grain breads instead of white bread or buns. If they've been raised this way, you should have no problem. But if they have already become accustomed to white bread and resist the change, you may have to alternate white and health breads until they learn to appreciate the difference. At least, when you make white-bread sandwiches, be sure to add more fiber to the filling. A tablespoon of bran can be slipped unobtrusively into almost any filling mixture.

Currant Nut Cheese Sandwiches

Use either Neufchâtel or farmers cheese (much lower in fat than cream cheese); soften to room temperature, then work in dried currants and chopped peanuts, ¼ cup each to 4 ounces (half an 8-ounce package) of cheese. Spread between sliced Boston brown bread or whole-wheat bread.

Raspberry Jam and Peanut Butter

Tastes best with oatmeal or cracked wheat bread. Spread one slice with peanut butter (preferably homemade or from a health store), the other with raspberry jam.

Apple Ham Sandwich Filling

Combine ½ cup of chopped unpeeled apple, 2 tablespoons of minced celery, 1½ tablespoons of mayonnaise (or ½ tablespoon of mayonnaise and 1 tablespoon of sour cream), a few drops of lemon juice, ½ cup of chopped ham, ½ teaspoon of prepared mustard. Makes ¾ cup. Good between whole-wheat bread.

Ham Peanut Sandwich Filling

Combine ⅓ cup of finely chopped cooked ham; ⅓ cup of finely chopped peanuts, ¼ cup of finely chopped celery, and ¼ cup of chopped pickle. Bind together with just enough mayonnaise to moisten. Makes a little less than 1 cup. Very good between slices of sour rye caraway bread.

Egg Nut Spread

1 celery stalk, trimmed	2 hard-cooked eggs
¼ cup broken walnut meats	2 tablespoons oil
1 medium carrot, scraped	Salt to taste

Feed ingredients into blender in order given, cutting carrot into cubes; beat until fairly smooth. Makes 1 cup. Good between sliced whole-wheat or sprouted wheat bread.

Nutty Cottage Cheese

Combine ½ cup of cottage cheese, 2 tablespoons of unsalted sunflower kernels, 2 tablespoons of whole-bran cereal, and 2 tablespoons of minced green pepper. Good between sliced Boston brown bread, whole-wheat, or any dark health bread.

Homemade Peanut Butter

1 pound shelled raw peanuts (available at health stores)
¼ cup wheat germ or bran meal
1 teaspoon salt, or to taste

1 tablespoon tahini sauce (sesame paste), also available at health stores, or 2 tablespoons oil and 1 teaspoon sesame seeds

Spread nuts out in a shallow pan, roast in oven set at 300° F., stirring several times, until nicely browned. Cool. Set aside about ¼ cup of nuts; put the rest in a blender with wheat germ, salt, and tahini (or oil and sesame seeds). Beat until smooth. Chop reserved nuts, stir in. Makes about 1 cup.

Peanut Date Butter

To ½ cup of peanut butter, add ½ cup of chopped dates and 1 teaspoon of bran meal. Blend well. Makes 1 cup.

Carrot Peanut Sandwich Filling

½ cup grated carrot
¼ cup bran meal
½ cup raw peanut butter
¼ cup coarsely chopped sunflower kernels

¼ cup dried currants or raisins
1 tablespoon margarine or softened butter

Combine all ingredients. Makes about 1½ cups. Can be used between whole-wheat or any health bread.

Tuna Salad Spread

1 can chunk-style tuna,
  drained
1 teaspoon horseradish
  (optional)
¼ cup chopped green pepper
¼ cup chopped celery

¼ cup grated carrot
1 tablespoon mayonnaise
1 tablespoon whole-bran
  cereal
¼ cup apple or pear, chopped
  fine

Combine all ingredients. Makes about 1¼ cups.

Nut Butter Spread

3 cups mixed nuts (almonds,
  hazelnuts, peanuts, walnuts, sunflower "nuts")
¼ cup toasted sesame seeds

¼ cup soft butter or
  margarine
1 teaspoon honey

Put nuts and seeds through medium blade of food grinder or
beat in blender—but they should still be "chunky." Add
butter, work to a paste. Sweeten with honey. Makes about 2
cups.

Vegetarian Salad Sandwich

1 cup shredded red or white
  cabbage, minced
¼ cup chopped dried apricots
¼ cup grated carrots

½ cup chopped red apples
2 tablespoons mayonnaise
2 tablespoons sour cream
Salt to taste

Combine ingredients, blend well. Makes about 1½ cups.

Baked Bean Sandwich

Mash cooked leftover baked beans, add a little catsup, a little
chopped celery and—optional—1 teaspoon of grated onion.
Best between white or oatmeal bread slices.

Pizzas and Crackers

Since pizzas have become such an integral part of the American way of life, they cannot be ignored, and if the dough is made from scratch, bran meal can be worked into it. When frozen pizza shells are used, add bran to the filling—it will not be noticeable in the taste of the sauce (if those who eat pizzas have any sensitivity to taste to begin with).

Hi-Fiber Pizza

1 envelope active dry yeast	2 tablespoons oil
1 cup warm (not hot) water	2½ cups all-purpose flour
	½ cup whole-wheat flour
1 teaspoon salt	½ cup pure bran meal

Dissolve yeast in lukewarm water. Stir in salt and olive oil; gradually add flour, beating after each addition. When dough is fairly stiff, add whole-wheat flour and bran meal, working into dough with fingers. Turn out on lightly floured board and knead until elastic (about 8 minutes). Place in greased 1-quart bowl; brush top with oil, cover lightly, let rise in warm protected place until doubled. Divide in half, roll each into a ball, then, with fingers, press to fit two 14-inch pizza pans, making edges thicker and slightly higher than center. Brush with more oil. Add filling. Bake in oven preheated to very hot (450° F.) for 20–25 minutes, or until crust is golden. Makes 2 pizzas or 16 servings. (One pizza shell may be frozen for future use, if desired. After shaping, place in freezer until hard, then remove from pan or sheet and wrap in plastic. Filling may also be frozen—everything but the cheese.)

PIZZA FILLING

2–3 tablespoons olive oil	¼ cup sunflower kernels or pine nuts
1 or 2 garlic cloves	
½ cup chopped onion	2 cups tomato sauce
2 tablespoons chopped parsley	2 tablespoons whole-bran cereal
¼ teaspoon oregano	16–20 pitted black olives
½ cup sliced mushrooms	Thin slices mozzarella cheese
¼ cup chopped green pepper	½ cup Parmesan cheese

Heat oil in frying pan, add garlic, onion, oregano, parsley, and mushrooms; sauté until soft and lightly browned—do not allow to burn. Add green pepper, sunflower kernels, tomato sauce, and bran; continue to cook over low heat until well blended (about 5 minutes longer). Spoon over prepared pizza shells. Top with black olives and the two kinds of cheese. Makes enough filling for 2 pizzas.

Since commercial crackers have little to offer except empty calories and chemicals, why not try making crackers at home? It's not hard—teen-agers could do it themselves.

Crispy Hi-Fiber Crackers

1½ cups quick-cooking oat- meal or steel-cut oats	¼ cup sesame or caraway seeds
1 cup whole-wheat flour	¼ cup shredded coconut
½ cup wheat germ	⅓ cup oil
½ teaspoon salt	½ cup water

Combine all dry ingredients in a mixing bowl, including sesame seeds and coconut. Beat in oil and water gradually to form a stiff dough. Roll or press out on a lightly greased or Teflon-coated baking sheet, making as thin as possible. (It will be easier if you cover the dough with waxed paper.) Cut in squares with the point of a sharp knife. Sprinkle with salt if desired. Bake in a slow oven (300° F.) for 30 minutes, or until golden brown. Cool before removing from baking sheet. Makes 3 dozen.

Whole-Wheat Sesame Crackers

6 tablespoons oil	½ teaspoon salt
½ cup water	½ cup sesame seeds
2 cups whole-wheat flour	

Beat oil and water together with egg beater or in blender until thickened. Add flour and salt, knead with fingers for a full 5 minutes, then let rest for 10 minutes. Divide mixture in half; roll out each half directly onto a greased or Teflon-coated baking sheet, as thin as possible. Sprinkle with sesame seeds and additional salt, and roll again with rolling pin, pressing seeds into the dough. Mark in squares and prick all over with a fork. Bake in oven preheated to 350° F. for 10 minutes, or until golden. Let cool before removing from pan. Repeat with second sheet of dough.

Nutritious High-Fiber Cookies

In addition to the recipes on the following pages, see Chapter 14 for more cookie recipes.

Bran Hermits

1 cup All-Bran cereal	½ cup regular margarine or
½ cup milk	butter
1 cup all-purpose flour	2 eggs
½ teaspoon baking soda	1 teaspoon vanilla flavoring
½ teaspoon cinnamon	½ cup coarsely chopped
¼ teaspoon nutmeg	peanuts
¼ teaspoon ginger	1 cup raisins or currants
1 cup firmly packed dark	
brown sugar	

Measure cereal and milk into small bowl; let stand until most of milk is absorbed. Sift together flour, soda, and spices. Set aside. Measure sugar and margarine into mixing bowl, beat until light and fluffy. Beat in eggs, vanilla, and cereal mixture. Add sifted dry ingredients and beat until all flour is moistened. Stir in peanuts and raisins. Drop by tablespoons onto lightly greased baking sheets about 2 inches apart. Bake in oven preheated to 375° F. for about 11 minutes, or until golden. Remove immediately from baking sheets. Cool on wire racks. Makes about 5 dozen.

Buckwheat Hermits

½ cup vegetable shortening
or oil
1 cup dark brown sugar or
light molasses
2 eggs, slightly beaten
¼ cup milk
1 teaspoon vanilla

1 teaspoon pumpkin pie
spice*
2 cups buckwheat pancake
mix
½ cup chopped raisins or
dates
½ cup chopped walnuts

Cream together shortening and sugar, or blend together oil and molasses. Add eggs, milk, and vanilla. Add spices to pancake mix, stir to blend thoroughly. Add to first mixture, blend the two. Stir in raisins and nuts. Drop by teaspoonfuls on greased baking sheet, 2 inches apart (they spread as they bake). Bake in oven preheated to 375° F. about 15 minutes until lightly browned around edges. Remove from baking sheet immediately to flat surface. They become more crisp as they cool. When cold, store in airtight container. Makes 4 dozen.

*Instead of pumpkin pie spice, use mixture of cinnamon, cloves and nutmeg.

Cocoa Drop Cookies

½ cup raisins, chopped
½ cup *hot* water
¼ cup 100% Bran cereal
½ cup (1 stick) margarine
¾ cup brown sugar
1 egg
½ cup buttermilk

1¾ cups all-purpose flour
½ teaspoon soda
½ teaspoon salt
½ cup Hershey's cocoa (not
a mix)
1 cup chopped nuts
(optional)

Soak raisins in hot water about 10 minutes; add cereal, let it stand until most of liquid is absorbed. Beat margarine until fluffy; beat in sugar, then egg and buttermilk. Combine flour, soda, salt, and cocoa. Add to creamed mixture alternately with raisin-bran mixture; beat just until flour is completely moistened. Stir in nuts. Chill for 1 hour, then drop by teaspoonfuls 2 inches apart on a greased or Teflon-coated baking sheet. Preheat oven to 400° F. before putting cookies in oven;

then bake 8–10 minutes, or until no imprint remains when lightly touched. Repeat until all batter is used. Makes 3–4 dozen.

Orange Carrot Cookies

1 cup oil or vegetable shortening
½ cup brown sugar
½ cup light molasses
2 eggs
1 cup unbleached flour
½ teaspoon baking powder
½ teaspoon baking soda
½ teaspoon salt
¼ teaspoon nutmeg
¼ teaspoon ground cloves
2 tablespoons grated orange peel
1 cup coarsely grated carrots
½ cup chopped peanuts
1½ cups crushed 40% Bran Flakes (crush before measuring)

Cream together oil or shortening and sugar, beat in molasses and eggs. Sift together unbleached flour, baking powder, soda, salt, and spices; add sugar mixture, orange rind, carrots, peanuts, and bran flakes; beat to mix thoroughly. Chill dough while preheating oven to 400° F. Drop mixture by teaspoonfuls on lightly greased or Teflon-coated baking sheet, 2 inches apart. Bake until no imprint remains when touched (10–12 minutes). Makes about 5 dozen.

Lacy Oatmeal Cookies

¾ cup vegetable shortening
1¼ cups packed dark brown sugar
1 egg
¼ cup apple juice
1 teaspoon vanilla
1 cup sifted all-purpose flour
1 teaspoon salt
½ teaspoon soda
3 cups rolled oats
½ cup slivered almonds

Beat together shortening and sugar until fluffy. Add egg, apple juice, and vanilla; beat until smooth. Sift together previously sifted flour, salt, and soda; add to first mixture. Stir in oats and nuts, blending thoroughly. Grease 1 or 2 baking sheets. Preheat oven to 350° F. Drop by teaspoonfuls 2 inches apart onto baking sheets. Bake until delicately browned (about 12 minutes). Repeat until all are baked. Makes 4–5 dozen.

Drinks

If your children eat plenty of fruit and vegetables, have whole-grain cereals for breakfast and sandwiches of whole-grain bread, they may not need bran sneaked into drinks. But if you have trouble getting them to eat anything but white bread, and you know they're getting too much candy, the extra bran suggested as an optional ingredient in some of the following drinks could be important for them.

Carob Eggnog

3 tablespoons instant carob   1 cup milk
  drink powder   1 egg
2 teaspoons whole-bran
  cereal

Put all ingredients in a blender and beat for 20 seconds. This makes a nutritious breakfast or after-school drink for youngsters. Makes 1 drink.

Carob Milk Shake

Follow the directions for Carob Eggnog but omit the egg.

Soy Nut Milk
(For those allergic to cow's milk)

1 cup soy milk powder   1 teaspoon honey
6 cups cold water
½ cup blanched toasted
  almonds

Combine ingredients in a blender and beat until smooth. Chill in refrigerator for 1 hour before serving. Can be used as a beverage, or to replace milk with cereals. Makes 1¾ quarts.

Carob Frosted

4 heaping teaspoons instant
  carob drink powder

1 cup cold milk
1 scoop coffee ice cream

Beat ingredients in blender about 30 seconds, or until smooth.
Makes 1 drink.

Hot Cocoa with Bran

1 tablespoon cocoa powder
  (not mix)
1 teaspoon whole-bran cereal
1 tablespoon brown sugar

¼ cup water
¾ cup milk
Cinnamon sticks, or dash of
  cinnamon

Combine cocoa powder and bran, sugar, and water. Heat,
stirring, until dissolved. Add milk, continue to cook until
heated through but do not allow to boil. Serve hot, stirring
with cinnamon stick, or dust cinnamon over top. Makes 1 drink.

Banana Coconut Frosted

¼ cup shredded dried
  coconut
1 small ripe banana

1 quart milk
1 teaspoon vanilla
½ cup vanilla ice cream
  (approx.)

Place coconut in blender, beat until very fine; add banana in
chunks, beat until mashed, then add part of the milk and
vanilla. Beat until smooth. Combine with remaining milk;
top each serving with a spoonful of ice cream. Makes 4 drinks.

Blueberry Frosted

1 cup blueberries
1 tablespoon sugar

1 quart whole milk
Scoop of vanilla ice cream

Beat blueberries and sugar in blender with 1 cup of milk until
foamy; combine with rest of milk, pour into glasses. Top each
serving with a spoonful of ice cream. Makes 4–6 tall drinks.

Strawberry Frosted

1 cup sliced fresh straw-
berries
1 tablespoon sugar, or
2 tablespoons whole-bran
cereal

1 quart cold milk
1 pint vanilla ice cream

If cereal is added to this drink, first soften it in milk, then combine with berries. Beat in blender until pureed, and add more milk, and part of the ice cream. If cereal is added, sugar is not necessary. Makes 6 drinks.

Orange Bran Nog

1 tablespoon whole-bran
cereal
¼ cup plain yogurt or whole
milk

1–1½ cups orange juice
1 egg
1 teaspoon vanilla
Dash of nutmeg

Combine cereal and yogurt or milk; let stand 5 minutes until softened, then add to remaining ingredients in blender and beat until foamy. Makes 1 serving.

Banana Nog

2 tablespoons whole-bran
cereal
2 cups milk
1 small ripe banana, cut in
chunks

1 egg
1 teaspoon vanilla

Soften cereal in milk. Beat banana to a puree in blender; add milk, egg, and vanilla, and beat until foamy. Makes 2 drinks.

Chapter 13

Desserts and Pastries

The conscientious follower of a high-fiber diet would skip pastries, puddings, and cakes entirely, settling on fruit for dessert, and preferably raw fruit from a fruit bowl, cut up with a knife and fork at the table in the European manner.

However, let's be realistic and face the fact that many Americans consider sweets the best part of the meal and, if denied them altogether, would sooner or later slip back into the old eating patterns.

Therefore I have tried to work out ways to reduce the sugar in popular desserts as much as possible and, in pastries, to offset the use of low-fiber white flour by adding bran meal either to the dough itself or to the filling.

I know it is possible to make delicious pastries entirely with whole-wheat flour—I've tasted some. But my own efforts to make whole-wheat pastry dough were such a dismal failure (and making pie crust has always been easy for me) that I concluded the easy way is to use a standard pastry recipe, working in the bran after the dough is already beginning to adhere. And, for fruit pies, I discovered that whole-bran cereal can be used both for part of the sweetener and as a thickener. While the pie is still warm, the graininess of the bran can be detected in the filling, but when cold, it tastes like any other filling. I recommend this especially for the lower-fiber fruits such as cherries, rhubarb, and peaches.

Fruit Desserts

Summer Compote

(LC)

Almost any combination of fresh seasonal fruits can be mixed with delicious results, but this is a sure winner: blackberries or red raspberries, sliced peaches, and blueberries. Instead of sugar, add reconstituted frozen tangerine juice.

Melon Delight

(LC)

For a large dinner party, cut a slice from the top side of a watermelon or honeydew, remove the seeds, and the fruit itself. Cut the melon into cubes or balls. Fill the inside with melon balls and other fruit, and sweeten with fruit juice and a little sherry or other sweet wine, if desired. Put the top back on, keep chilled in the refrigerator until time to serve, and use the melon shell as a serving dish.

Blueberries and Yogurt

(LC)

Either fresh blueberries or the frozen whole (unsweetened) blueberries may be used for this dessert. Add 1 tablespoon of honey and ¼ teaspoon of cinnamon to 1 cup of plain yogurt. Stir the yogurt through the berries and marinate in the refrigerator for 1 hour before serving.

Winter Compote

(LC)

Defrost frozen red raspberries, drain off the syrup (save all but ¼ cup of it for sweetening other fruits), and combine berries with canned pear halves and whole blueberries (fresh or frozen and defrosted). Serve topped with coconut or toasted almonds.

Figs in Orange Juice

Marinate dried figs in orange juice to cover for 24–48 hours. Add a little lemon juice shortly before serving. (Another way is to marinate the figs in dry white wine.)

Baked Apples with Raisins

Core large baking apples (1 to a serving), place in baking dish, and spoon a few raisins in the cavity of each. Dribble in about ½ teaspoon of honey in each. Bake in moderate to hot oven for 40 minutes, or until skin has begun to burst. Serve either warm or cold, topped with sour cream or yogurt.

Diced Dried Fruit Compote

½ cup chopped dates
½ cup chopped dried apricots
½ cup chopped dried pears (optional)
6 large pitted softened prunes, chopped

3 canned peach halves, chopped
¼ cup canned peach syrup

Combine all ingredients and marinate together overnight. Serve this way, or top with yogurt blended with honey to taste. Makes about 8 servings.

Yogurt Sundae

(LC)

Top raspberry-flavored yogurt with sliced fresh or canned peaches, blueberries, and toasted soybeans.

Baked Meringue-Topped Peaches

4 large fresh peaches
1 tablespoon sherry
½ cup blanched almonds, chopped
¼ cup wheat germ

¼ cup honey
2 eggs, separated
1 tablespoon confectioner's sugar

Scald peaches to loosen skins (though if fully ripe, the skins should come off easily with a sharp paring knife). Cut each in half, remove pits and scoop out a little of the fruit to make a deep hollow in each. Sprinkle with sherry. Combine almonds, wheat germ, honey, and the yolks of the eggs. Place the 8 peach halves, hollow side up, in a shallow baking dish with a cover. Spoon almond mixture into the peach halves. This can be done ahead, but cover pan or baking dish with plastic wrap and refrigerate it. About 40 minutes before dinner is to be served, preheat oven to 375° F., bake peaches, covered, for 20 minutes. Meanwhile beat egg whites to a stiff meringue and fold in confectioner's sugar. Remove baking dish from oven, uncover, pile meringue over peach halves and return to oven, reducing temperature to 325° F., until meringue is lightly browned. Serve warm but not hot. Makes 4 servings, 2 peach halves to each serving.

Peach Pear Compote

When peaches and pears are in season, try this compote. Dip fruit in scalding water to soften skins, then peel off. Cut in halves to remove pits or seeds (or leave whole, if preferred). Heat together in kettle 1 cup of sugar and 3 cups of water; when boiling, add 1 whole lemon, thinly sliced, and 4 or 5 pieces of fruit at a time—do not crowd. Simmer about 10 minutes; remove with slotted spoon, add more fruit. When all are cooked, cover in bowl with remaining syrup; chill. The syrup tastes as if it were part wine, and the amount of sugar per serving is quite small.

Sugarless Sweeteners for Fresh Fruit Salad

Instead of adding sugar to fresh cut-up fruit, add chopped pitted dates, chopped raisins, unsweetened shredded coconut, and/or unsweetened fruit juice (canned pineapple, tangerine, or apple juice, or syrup from canned dietetic pack fruit). Or a tablespoon or two of sherry or another sweet wine may be added. Marinate fruit mixture for at least an hour before serving.

Raspberry Parfait

1 teaspoon unflavored gelatin
¼ cup water
1 10-ounce package frozen
   raspberries, thawed

½ cup sour cream or thick
   plain yogurt

Sprinkle gelatin over water in a small bowl to soften, then place bowl over hot water in large saucepan and stir until gelatin is dissolved. Stir gelatin into thawed raspberries (with their syrup) and chill until mixture starts to set (about 20 minutes). Layer raspberries with sour cream in four parfait glasses, with the cream on top. Chill for 1–2 hours. Makes 4 servings.

Frozen Banana Dessert

(LC)

2 large fully ripe bananas,
   peeled
½ cup plain yogurt (whole-
   milk type)

2 tablespoons wildflower
   honey
1 teaspoon vanilla

The simplest way to serve this dessert is to cut each of the bananas in half, wrap loosely in foil, then place in freezer and allow to freeze completely. Blend together yogurt, honey, and vanilla and serve as a dip or topping for the frozen banana. Serves 2.

Another way is to mash the bananas first, add the yogurt, honey, and vanilla, and freeze in an ice tray, then serve in sherbets, topped with wheat germ, crushed nuts, chopped candied orange peel, or chopped dates. The surprise is what banana tastes like when frozen: almost like banana cream.

(Still another way is to freeze the bananas, cut in slices while still frozen, and dribble honey over the top; serve yogurt on the side.)

Apricot Yogurt

(LC)

Combine 1 pint of plain or vanilla yogurt with 1 tablespoon of molasses, ⅓ cup of chopped dried apricots, and 1 tablespoon of buckwheat grains. Chill for 1 hour before serving.

Ice Cream Desserts

Ice creams manufactured without fillers (gelatin or vegetable gum or both) are more expensive but also a far better product. On the other hand, the cheaper ice creams are made with milk, some with instant dry milk powder, and therefore contain less fat. But all are high in sucrose!

Nevertheless, ice creams, like steaks and pizzas, are so much a part of the American way of life that we might as well "improve" them with fiber and not try to eliminate them entirely from the scene.

Easy Ice Cream Sundae

Top each serving of ice cream with a spoonful of frozen (thawed) raspberries and sprinkle with chopped nuts, wheat germ, or Wheat Chex.

Carob Banana Split

For each serving arrange in a dessert dish 2 lengthwise quarters of bananas. Add a scoop of vanilla or coffee ice cream, dribble honey or pure maple syrup over the ice cream, and top with carob nuggets. Add chopped nuts, too, if you want to go all the way.

Hi-Fiber Fruit Nut Sundae

Top each serving of ice cream with any of these fruits: chopped dates, sweetened blackberries, fresh sliced strawberries, or blueberries. Use as topping or stir into the ice cream any of these: chopped peanuts, sunflower kernels (the salted kind), toasted slivered almonds, or toasted soybeans. Or, instead of nuts or seeds, top the sundaes with wheat germ, whole-bran cereal, or crumbled Wheat Chex.

Carob Syrup

1 cup carob powder (not a mix)	½ teaspoon salt
	¼ cup brown sugar
1 tablespoon cornstarch or arrowroot	2 cups water
	2 teaspoons vanilla

Make sure you use the plain carob powder, not the drink mix. Combine powder with cornstarch, salt, and sugar. Gradually add water, bring to a boil, and boil gently for 5 minutes. Stir frequently. Remove from heat, cool 5 minutes, add vanilla. Store in refrigerator to use as wanted over ice cream or puddings. Also good over canned pears. Makes 2 cups.

Crunchy Ice Cream Topping

4 tablespoons butter or margarine	¼ cup crushed whole-bran cereal
¼ cup dark brown sugar	1 cup Wheat Chex crushed to ½ cup
1 cup rolled oats	
1 tablespoon buckwheat grains	¾ cup unsweetened shredded coconut

Melt butter, add sugar, and stir until well blended. Stir in remaining ingredients and cook and stir over low heat until lightly browned (about 10 minutes). Cool for 15 minutes, then break into pieces. Chill to use when wanted as topping for ice cream, fresh fruit, or puddings. Makes 2 cups.

Pies and Pie Crusts

Since many millions of frozen pie shells are sold daily in supermarkets, and I know how many home cooks look on rolling out pie crust as a formidable task, I tried to develop ways to add fiber to ready-to-bake pie shells. After several unsuccessful attempts, I concluded it would be better to add fiber to the filling in one way or another, as has been done in several of the following recipes. The best of the pie crust recipes, in my estimation, is the one immediately following, which has bran meal worked into the dough, with unbleached white flour as the base.

Hi-Fiber Pie Crust I
(for 2-crust pie)

1½ cups unbleached all-
   purpose flour
½ teaspoon salt
½ cup vegetable shortening

¼ cup water
2–3 tablespoons pure bran
   meal

Place flour and salt in mixing bowl and stir to blend well. Cut in shortening with table knife until the size of peas or smaller. Add water, about a teaspoon at a time, tossing with a fork to blend. Pick up dough with hands and knead just enough to hold together. Work in bran meal with fingers as you continue to knead it into a ball. Cut dough in half; roll out on lightly floured board, one half at a time, to 10 inches in diameter (for a 9-inch pie pan). Place lower crust in pan, overlapping edges; cut with knife around rim. Moisten edges with water.

Roll out second crust. Fold over, cut slits in center. Add filling to pie and place top crust over filling. Press edges together with tines of fork. Then trim edges with a quarter-inch overlap and flute upright with fingers. Prick top of crust with fork. Bake in oven *preheated* to 400° F. until crust is golden brown (about 45 minutes). Filling should be bubbling through the slits. (The bran gives the crust a brownish hue but is crisp and delicious.)

Hi-Fiber Pie Crust II
(for 1-crust pie)

1 cup unbleached all-
   purpose flour
¼ teaspoon salt
⅓ cup vegetable shortening

2–3 tablespoons water
1–2 tablespoons pure bran
   meal

Proceed as for 2-crust pastry (in previous recipe). Fit into pie pan, pushing down with fingers so that it fits like a glove (it will shrink a little during baking) and so that the rim stands up well around edges. Prick bottom with a fork to lessen shrinking. If it is to be used as a baked shell, bake in oven preheated to 425° until golden (15–20 minutes). If it is to be unbaked before filling is added, brush unbeaten egg white over bottom so that filling will not make crust soggy, and place in freezer for 5 minutes before baking. This helps to brown the pastry before the melting fat causes the rim to wobble over.

Apple Date Pie

Hi-Fiber Pastry for 2-crust pie
2 or 3 firm tart apples
4 pitted dates, cut in pieces
1 teaspoon lemon juice
½ teaspoon grated lemon rind
3–4 tablespoons sugar (white or brown)

Prepare pastry as described. For filling, do not peel apples, only core them and cut away any soft spots. Add enough apples to fill the pie pan to the brim. Scatter pieces of dates through the apples. Sprinkle with lemon juice and grated rind. Add sugar and cover with top crust. Bake at 400° F. (in preheated oven) for 45 minutes. Because apples are not high in moisture, you may not see juice bubbling up through the slits, but if your oven is accurate, this should be ample baking time. Makes 1 pie, or 6 servings.

Apple Prune Pie

Use pitted prunes instead of dates, in the same measure.

Blueberry Pie I

Hi-Fiber Pastry for 2-crust pie
1 pint fresh blueberries, or a 10-ounce package frozen whole (unsweetened) blueberries
1 tablespoon soy or soya carob flour
⅓–½ cup sugar
Grated lemon rind and 1 teaspoon lemon juice

Prepare pastry and roll out to fit an 8-inch pie pan. Combine blueberries, flour, and sugar; stir in grated lemon rind and juice. Place in prepared bottom pastry, top with second crust, and bake in preheated 400° F. oven until crust is golden and sauce bubbling. Makes 1 pie.

Blueberry Pie II

Pastry for 2-crust pie
(pastry mix or 2 frozen
commercial pie shells)
1 pint fresh blueberries, or a
10-ounce package frozen
whole blueberries, thawed

½ cup Kellogg's Bran Buds
2 tablespoons sugar
Grated lemon rind and
1 teaspoon lemon juice

Prepare pastry with piecrust mix according to package directions; or use frozen commercial pie shells. Mix together the blueberries, bran, sugar, grated lemon rind and juice. Place in lower crust, moisten rim of pastry, then cover with upper crust, with slits cut in center. Press edges together with tines of fork. Bake in preheated 400° F. oven for 45 minutes, or until crust is golden. The thickened filling is not likely to be bubbling, so don't worry. Let pie cool completely before cutting. Makes one 8-inch pie.

The preceding recipe may be used for any fruit pie, but the amount of sugar needed will vary according to the fruit. Tart (sour) red cherries will require ⅔ cup of sugar, and rhubarb may require more. As a general rule, consider ½ cup of the bran cereal as containing the equivalent of 3 tablespoons of sugar, and since the bran itself has natural sweetness, the normal sugar measure may be reduced by ⅓ cup. The bran also serves as a thickener, so no flour or cornstarch is needed, which some fruit pie recipes require.

Caramel Custard Pie

Unbaked pie shell for
1-crust 9-inch pie
2 tablespoons soft butter
or margarine
¼ cup Kellogg's Bran Buds
1 tablespoon dark brown
sugar

3 eggs
1 tablespoon honey
⅛ teaspoon salt
1¾ cups milk
½ teaspoon vanilla
⅛ teaspoon nutmeg

Line a Pyrex pie pan with pastry, fluting the edges. (Piecrust mix may be used to make the pastry, but a commercial ready-to-use pie shell is not recommended—it is too skimpy to hold the custard mixture.) Combine butter or margarine, bran, and brown sugar. Distribute mixture as evenly as possible over bottom of crust, pressing down with fork.

Beat eggs until no white shows, but not until foamy. Heat together the honey, salt, milk, and vanilla, just until honey is well blended with milk. Add to eggs; add nutmeg.

Preheat oven to 400° F. Place pastry shell with bran mixture over bottom in oven for 5 minutes, until mixture begins to bubble. Remove from oven, add custard mixture, return to oven, and turn down heat to 325° F. Bake about 50 minutes, or until knife inserted in center comes out clean. Bran mixture will rise to top, giving it a golden crust. (The filling falls as it cools, but it has delicious flavor.)

In colonial times, bean pie was both a New England and a Southern pastry. It can be made with peabeans or pinto beans, but when made with black beans, it has a chocolatey appearance and it tastes much like moist gingerbread in a pastry crust. The beans must be cooked until very, very soft, however. It should be served warm, topped with sour cream or whipped sweet cream. This is an excellent dessert for active growing children.

Black Bean Pie

Unbaked Hi-Fiber Crust for a 9-inch pie
2 cups cooked black beans (1 cup before soaking)
½ cup raisins
1 tablespoon cornstarch
¼ cup apple juice
½ cup milk
½ teaspoon nutmeg
½ teaspoon cinnamon
⅓ cup light molasses
2 eggs, beaten

The night before, pour boiling water over beans, bring water again to a boil, then turn off heat and soak overnight. Soak raisins in hot water. Next day, add 1 teaspoon of salt and more water to cover beans 1 inch. Simmer covered until very tender (on top of stove, in oven at 325° F., or in crock-pot, or try cooking them in a pressure cooker).

When beans are tender, puree in blender or force through food mill. Measure; use a little less than 2 cups. Add remaining ingredients in order given.

Prepare pastry and fit into Pyrex pan, fluting edges high around rim. Preheat oven to 400° F. Pour bean mixture into unbaked crust, bake for 10 minutes at 400° F., then reduce to 325°. Bake until knife inserted in center comes out clean (about 35 minutes longer). Cool to room temperature but, if possible, serve before completely cold. Very rich and filling. Makes 1 large pie.

Pecan Pumpkin Pie

Hi-Fiber Pastry for 1-crust pie
2 cups cooked or canned pumpkin
3 eggs, slightly beaten
½ cup sugar
½ cup light molasses
¼ teaspoon ground ginger
½ teaspoon cinnamon
½ teaspoon nutmeg
¼ teaspoon crushed cardamom or cloves
¾ cup half-and-half
¼ cup brandy*
43 pecan halves

Prepare pastry, rolling out to 10 inches in diameter. Flute edges of pie high around rim (patch edges with scraps of pastry, if necessary). Place pastry in freezer while preparing filling and, at the same time, preheat oven to 400° F.

Combine pumpkin, eggs, sugar, molasses, spices, cream, and brandy. Pour into chilled pie shell. Bake for 5 minutes, reduce heat to 350° F., bake about 40 minutes longer, or until knife inserted in center comes out clean. Cool completely before cutting. Makes one 9-inch pie.

*If preferred, use 1 cup of half-and-half and omit the brandy.

Pumpkin Banana Pie

As a way to reduce somewhat the total calorie and sugar content in the above, use 1 cup of pumpkin and 1 cup of mashed banana; *omit the sugar,* so that only ½ cup of molasses is added for sweetening. Add the pecans or not, as your conscience dictates. Pecans are a good source of fiber, but unfortunately also of fat.

Carob Meringue Pie

1 baked pie shell, or Coconut Oat Crust	¼ teaspoon salt
⅓ cup carob powder	2¼ cups milk
¼ cup sugar	1 teaspoon vanilla
3 tablespoons cornstarch or arrowroot	3 eggs, separated
	1 tablespoon confectioner's sugar

Prepare pie shell. Combine carob powder, sugar, cornstarch, and salt; stir in milk and vanilla, and the egg yolks. Cook in top of double boiler or over very low heat, stirring almost continuously, until thickened. Remove from heat, cool in pan for 5 minutes, then stir to remove film over top and pour into pie shell. Beat egg whites until stiff; stir in confectioner's sugar without breaking foam. Pile over filling; bake in slow oven (325° F.) until meringue is golden. This is so much like chocolate pie, it can pass as the same (though the texture is slightly more granular), and it is both lower in calories (and fat) and higher in fiber than chocolate. Makes 1 pie.

Coconut Oat Crust

1 cup rolled oats	½ cup flaked coconut
3 tablespoons packed brown sugar	¼ cup slivered almonds, coarsely crushed pecans, or chopped sunflower kernels
3–4 tablespoons butter or margarine, melted	

Combine ingredients, press into bottom and up sides of an 8- or 9-inch pie pan. Bake in moderate (350° F.) oven for 8 minutes, or until golden. Remove, cool to room temperature, then chill. Makes 1 crust.

Crunchy Bran Crust

Instead of oats in previous recipe, use crushed 40% Bran Flakes or Shredded Wheat plus 1 teaspoon of bran meal.

Almond Triscuit Crust

1¾ cups Triscuits, crushed
    to 1 cup
½ cup blanched almonds,
    crushed to ¼ cup

¼ cup brown sugar, packed
3 tablespoons melted butter
    or margarine

Prepare as directed for Coconut Oat Crust.

Wheat Chex Almond Crust

Instead of Triscuits in above recipe, use 2 cups of Wheat Chex crushed to 1 cup.

Lemon Chiffon Pie

Almond Triscuit Crust
1 envelope unflavored
    gelatin
¼ cup cold water
3 eggs, separated
½ cup sugar

⅓ cup fresh lemon juice
½ teaspoon salt
Grated rind of ½ lemon
¼ cup chopped walnuts
¼ cup crushed 40% Bran
    Flakes

Prepare crust as directed; chill. Soften gelatin in cold water in 1-quart mixing bowl. Place in top of double boiler the egg yolks, sugar, lemon juice, and salt. Stir over hot, not boiling, water until mixture thickens. Remove from heat; add to softened gelatin, stir until dissolved. Stir in grated lemon rind. Chill until mixture is consistency of unbeaten egg whites; beat until fluffy. Separately beat egg whites (with clean rotary beater) until stiff; fold into gelatin mixture. Pile filling into baked chilled crust; sprinkle mixture of nuts and cereal over top. Chill until firm. Makes 6 servings.

Pumpkin Chiffon Pie

Coconut Oat Crust
1 envelope unflavored gelatin
¼ cup cold water
½ cup packed brown sugar
½ teaspoon salt
1½ teaspoons pumpkin pie spice

2 egg yolks, beaten
1 cup whole milk
1 cup canned pumpkin
¼ cup brandy or rum or 1 teaspoon vanilla
2 egg whites
Whipped cream (optional)

Prepare Coconut Oat Crust. For filling, dissolve gelatin in cold water; add sugar, salt, spices, egg yolks, milk, and pumpkin. Place mixture in heavy saucepan over low heat and stir constantly until thoroughly heated. Remove from heat, stir in brandy or rum. Cool, then chill until mixture has become syrupy in consistency.

Beat egg whites until stiff; fold beaten whites into pumpkin mixture. Spoon into chilled crust. Keep refrigerated until time to serve. Serve garnished with whipped cream, if desired. Makes 1 pie.

Instant Ice Cream Pie

Use any of the crumb mixtures for an "instant" crust, fill the baked chilled crumb crust with ice cream, top with fresh fruit. Make it a Peach Melba Pie by topping vanilla ice cream with sliced fresh peaches, and over the peaches spoon thawed frozen red raspberries with part of the raspberry syrup.

Torta di Ricotta

Almond Triscuit Crust
1 pound (16 ounces) ricotta cheese
¼ cup honey
¼ cup chopped dates
1 cup crushed toasted almonds

4 eggs
Grated rind of 1 lemon
Pinch of salt
¼ cup crushed Triscuits

Prepare crust, bake, and chill. Force cheese through sieve or beat in blender until very smooth. Stir in honey, dates, and ¾ cup of the almonds. Beat in eggs, one at a time, finally adding lemon rind and salt. Combine remaining ¼ cup of crushed almonds with crushed Triscuits; spread over top. Bake at 350° F. about 40 minutes, or until knife inserted in center comes out clean. Cool. Cut into 8 wedges (filling is very rich). Makes 8 servings.

Cakes

It is hard indeed to make a cake without using much sugar, and without refined white flour. Dedicated cake lovers will not drool over any of the following, but children should be happy with them, and so should most grown-ups.

Carrot Cake

1 stick (¼ pound) butter or margarine, softened	½ teaspoon cinnamon
1 cup dark brown sugar*	1 cup *hot* water
1 egg	1 cup coarsely grated raw carrots
2¾ cups whole-wheat flour	1 teaspoon grated lemon rind
2 teaspoons baking soda	
½ teaspoon salt	1 teaspoon lemon juice

Grease, then flour an 8x8x2-inch baking pan. Beat together butter and sugar until fluffy. Add egg and blend well. Combine flour with soda, salt, and cinnamon; add to butter-sugar mixture alternately with hot water. Stir in carrots, lemon rind, and juice. Pour into prepared baking pan and bake in oven preheated to 350° F. for 1 hour, or until cake tester comes out clean. Let cool in pan for 10 minutes, then turn out on rack. Serve topped with whipped cream, ice cream, or with yogurt blended with just enough molasses to sweeten. Makes 9 or 10 servings. (This is a gingerbread-type cake, very moist, amazingly good.)

*Or use ½ cup each of brown sugar and molasses.

Bran Molasses Cake

1 cup unbleached all-purpose flour
1 teaspoon baking powder
½ teaspoon baking soda
½ teaspoon salt
1 cup All Bran or Bran Buds

1 cup milk
½ cup molasses
1 egg
¼ cup shortening
½ cup chopped pitted dates

Stir together flour, baking powder, soda, and salt. Set aside. In large mixing bowl, combine the cereal, milk, and molasses. Let stand until most of liquid is absorbed. Add egg and shortening. Beat well. Stir in dates. Add dry ingredients, stirring only until well mixed. Spread in greased 8x8x2-inch baking pan.

Bake in oven preheated to 400° F. about 20 minutes, or until cake tester inserted in center comes out clean. Cut into squares. Serve warm or cool, topped with whipped cream or ice cream.

Old-Fashioned Gingerbread

1 cup dark unsulfured molasses
1 cup boiling water
½ cup vegetable shortening
1 egg, beaten
2 cups rye flour, or 1 cup rye flour, 1 cup whole wheat flour

1 teaspoon baking soda
1 teaspoon salt
1 teaspoon ginger
1 teaspoon cinnamon
½ teaspoon cloves

Grease and flour an 8x8-inch baking pan. Combine molasses and boiling water, add shortening, stir until melted. Add egg. Combine flour (or flours), baking soda, salt, and spices. Add molasses mixture, stirring just until all flour is moistened; pour batter into pan, shake pan to level batter. Bake in oven set at 325° for 45–50 minutes until a toothpick inserted in the center comes out clean. Cut into squares while in pan. Best served warm, right out of the oven, topped with whipped cream or ice cream, or with canned peaches topped with yogurt-molasses mixture (1 teaspoon of molasses to 1 cup of yogurt—or sour cream). Also a good after-school snack. Makes about nine 3-inch squares.

Puddings and Baked Fruit Desserts

Veiled Country Lass
(Danish Apple Cake)

4 cups soft crumbs of 100 percent rye bread
¼ pound (1 stick) butter
2 tablespoons sugar

2 cups smooth applesauce
¼ cup red raspberry jam
¼ cup currant jelly
½ cup heavy cream, whipped

Remove crusts from bread, break into fine pieces. Melt butter (or margarine) in frying pan, add crumbs and sugar; stir over high heat until crumbs are crisp and lightly browned. Spoon half the crumbs over center of round platter (10 inch). Spoon thin layer of applesauce over crumbs, then add remaining crumbs and remaining applesauce in layers. With flat side of knife, mold into cake shape. Chill for 1 hour or longer. Heat jam and jelly together, stirring constantly, until melted. Remove from heat; cool. After cake has chilled, again press into shape with knife blade; spread jam mixture over top, then frost sides of cake with whipped cream. Keep chilled until time to serve. Makes 4–6 servings.

Apple Bran Betty

3 cups sliced (not peeled) apples
1 cup crushed 40% Bran Flakes
2 tablespoons crushed whole-bran cereal
1 tablespoon brown sugar

½ teaspoon cinnamon
Pinch of salt
1 teaspoon grated lemon rind
1 tablespoon lemon juice
2 tablespoons butter
¼ cup hot water

Prepare apples. In a separate bowl, combine all remaining ingredients except butter and water. (The bran cereals should be measured *after* crushing.) Arrange apples in layers with cereal mixture in a buttered 1-quart baking dish, with cereal mixture on top. Add butter to water, pour mixture over top. Bake uncovered in oven preheated to 350° F. until top is browned (35–40 minutes). Serve warm with cream or ice cream. Makes 6 servings.

Fruit Crisp
(Basic Recipe)

4 cups fresh fruit*
½ cup (1 stick) butter or margarine
½ cup brown sugar
¼ cup soy or whole-wheat flour
½ teaspoon cinnamon
1–1¼ cups 40% Bran Flakes, or rolled oats, or a mixture of the two

Arrange fruit in a shallow buttered baking dish. Beat together butter, sugar, flour, and cinnamon. Stir in cereal or cereals. (Instead of bran, Shredded Wheat or Wheat Chex may be used.) Sprinkle mixture over fruit. Bake at 375° F. for 25–30 minutes. Serve warm, topped with cream or ice cream. Makes 8 servings.

*Fruits which may be used include apples, blackberries, blueberries, fresh peaches, and rhubarb. However, for rhubarb, more sugar will be needed, perhaps as much as ½ cup more.

Blackberry Slump

¾ cup dark brown sugar
¼ teaspoon nutmeg
¼ teaspoon cinnamon
8 slices whole-wheat or other whole-grain bread
½ cup (1 stick) butter or
margarine, melted
4 cups fresh blackberries, washed, picked over
1 teaspoon lemon juice
½ teaspoon grated lemon peel

Grease a 9x5x3-inch loaf pan. Blend together sugar and spices. Cut bread into strips. Place ⅓ of the strips in bottom of pan, sprinkle with 2 tablespoons of sugar-spice mixture, add half the berries, sprinkle them with lemon juice and grated rind and 2 tablespoons of sugar-spice mixture. Repeat, with bread as top layer. Preheat oven to 375° F. Cover pan tightly with foil during first 15 minutes (allowing juice to form), then uncover and, with fork, press top layer of bread down so it is partially covered with juice. Continue baking another 20–25 minutes until juice is bubbling and bread lightly toasted. Serve warm with cream or ice cream. Makes 6 servings.

Blueberry Slump

Use 4 cups of blueberries and oatmeal bread in above recipe.

Red Raspberry Slump

This you can make any time of year with frozen raspberries. Use two 10-ounce packages with their syrup; decrease sugar in above recipe to ¼ cup, omit spices, and use oatmeal or cracked wheat bread. Before starting to bake, press bread down with back of spoon so as to be covered with juice. Pan need not be covered.

Plum Pudding
(for 1-quart steam mold)

¾ cup whole-wheat or rye flour	¾ cup currants
½ teaspoon soda	½ cup slivered candied lemon or orange peel
¼ teaspoon salt	
¼ teaspoon cinnamon	1 cup soft whole-wheat breadcrumbs, in fine pieces
¼ teaspoon nutmeg	
½ teaspoon crushed cardamom	¾ cup finely chopped beef suet
¾ cup chopped pitted prunes or dates	½ cup molasses
	2 eggs, beaten
	¼ cup brandy*

First prepare steam mold. Recipe will exactly fit a 1-quart steam mold with cover, or 2 metal cans (1 pound size) may be used, the tops carefully removed with a can opener. Grease insides generously.

Combine flour, soda, salt, and spices. Add fruit, toss to cover with flour. Add remaining ingredients in order given,

*Instead of brandy, unsweetened apple juice may be used.

blending thoroughly. Spoon into mold or metal cans. Cover with fitted cover, or put brown paper over top, greased on the inside, and secure in place with large rubber bands or tie with butcher's cord. Place on rack inside large kettle, with water three-quarters of the way up the sides. Bring to a boil and keep simmering for 4 hours. Cool on rack. Do not attempt to turn out of mold (or metal cans) until cold. Then loosen from sides with a thin-bladed knife. To reheat, replace in buttered mold and heat in simmering water. Serve hot, with hard sauce. Makes 6–8 rich servings.

Hard Sauce

Beat together 3 tablespoons of softened butter and ½ cup of confectioner's sugar. Chill.

Banana Bread Pudding

2 cups milk	½ cup currants or raisins
1 cup mashed banana	1 teaspoon grated lemon rind
⅓ cup brown sugar	4 slices whole-wheat or
½ teaspoon salt	oatmeal bread, each slice
2 eggs, slightly beaten	cut in thirds

Heat milk to scalding; stir in banana, sugar, and salt. Cool slightly. Add mixture to eggs; add remaining ingredients and pour into greased baking dish. Bake at 350° F. for 50 minutes, or until knife inserted near center comes out clean. Let stand for 15 minutes before serving.

Peach Bread Pudding

Instead of bananas, use 1 cup of cut-up fresh peaches; add sugar to peaches before mixing with milk.

Indian Pudding

6 cups (1½ quarts) milk	½ cup dark molasses
½ cup stone-ground yellow	½ teaspoon salt
cornmeal	½ teaspoon ground ginger
1 tablespoon butter	½ cup currants or raisins

Heat 2 cups of the milk to scalding; gradually stir in corn-meal and butter, stirring constantly over low heat until thickened. Add 2 cups of cold milk, plus molasses, salt, and ginger. Pour into buttered 2½-quart baking dish. Place in oven set at 275° F. Bake for 1 hour, stirring once or twice; then add 1 cup more of milk. Bake another hour; stir once or twice during the hour, and add remaining milk and fruit. Continue to bake, stirring occasionally, for 2 hours longer. The pudding will look curdled in the beginning, but as it bakes down, it becomes smooth and creamy. This sounds like a lot of trouble, but it's the kind of thing you can enjoy doing on a winter day when you want to stay indoors all day any-way. And it makes a marvelous dessert. Best served warm, topped with cream or ice cream. Makes 8–10 servings.

Kadaife
(Greek Dessert)

4 large Shredded Wheat biscuits	2 tablespoons sugar
1 cup milk	1 egg, beaten
1 cup chopped almonds or pistachios	1 teaspoon cinnamon
	¼ cup butter, melted

Lightly grease an 8-inch-square baking dish. Soften Shredded Wheat in milk. Place biscuits in dish, spread mixture of nuts, sugar, egg, and cinnamon over top. Pack down with back of spoon. Pour melted butter over top. Bake in oven pre-heated to 375° F. until top is golden and crisp (about 30 minutes). Remove. Prepare Syrup (see below). Pour Syrup over baked biscuits. Cool completely before serving. Makes 6–8 servings.

Kadaife Syrup

Combine in saucepan ½ cup of sugar, 1 cup of water, ¼ tea-spoon of cloves, ¼ teaspoon of cinnamon, and a long strip of thinly peeled orange rind. Bring to a boil, cook until syrup begins to thread. Remove orange rind before pouring syrup over biscuits.

Apricot Prune Coffee Cake

DOUGH:

1 package active dry yeast
¼ cup lukewarm water
½ cup milk
2 tablespoons honey or brown sugar
¼ teaspoon salt

¼ cup shortening
2–2½ cups unbleached flour
2 eggs, beaten
½ cup finely crushed all-bran cereal or bran meal

TOPPING:

1 pound pitted prunes
1 cup dried apricots
2 tablespoons buckwheat grains
½ cup sunflower kernels or dry-roasted peanuts

2 tablespoons dark brown sugar
2 tablespoons softened butter
1 teaspoon cinnamon

Soften yeast in lukewarm water. Heat milk to scalding; add honey or brown sugar, salt, and shortening. Cool to luke-warm. Add to milk about 1 cup of the flour to make a thick batter. Stir in yeast, then eggs, blend well. Add remaining flour, enough to make a soft, pliable dough. Turn out on lightly floured board and knead until smooth and shiny; work in bran as you knead for about 10 minutes. Put in large greased bowl, turning so all sides are greased. Cover, let rise in warm protected place until doubled. Punch down, let rest for 10 minutes, then shape to fit a 9x9-inch-square greased baking pan or a 1-quart ring mold. Allow to rise again until doubled.

Pour boiling water over prunes and apricots to soften, but do not cook. Drain thoroughly.

Arrange rows of prunes and apricots over top of dough, sprinkling buckwheat and sunflower kernels (or peanuts) around the fruit. Combine sugar, butter, and cinnamon; sprinkle mixture over top of fruit. Bake in oven preheated to 350° F. for 30–40 minutes until golden.

CHAPTER 14

Gifts to Make
for Those You Love

There are many times of the year when a homemade gift becomes a special way of saying you care; a gift of food is always appreciated.

Some of the following, I'm afraid, use quite large quantities of sugar or honey, though they also incorporate valuable high-fiber ingredients. One that requires no sugar at all is the Cranberry Coconut Relish which I created to prove a relish can be made without sugar. If it is made as a molded salad, it must be carried by hand to the recipient and promptly refrigerated, but then most food gifts are delivered by hand anyway.

Another gift idea is to make up a granola mixture (using one of the combinations suggested in Chapter 4, or your own invention) and package it in plastic bags, placed inside decorated plastic food containers.

Shredded dried coconut also makes a good gift. In the winter months, fresh coconuts often can be found in the supermarkets; the following recipe shows how easy it is to shred and dry your own. Coconut will keep almost indefinitely in a covered jar on the shelf; it requires no refrigeration (unlike the commercial product) and no sweetening.

To Open a Fresh Coconut

First punch holes in the three eyes of the coconut, using an icepick or screwdriver and hammer. Pour out and save coconut liquid (if the coconut is still fresh, the liquid is sweet enough to drink, or it can be used in recipes for coconut milk). Bake unopened coconut in the oven (350° F.) about ½ hour, or at 300° F. for 1 hour, until the shell is noticeably browner, perhaps even a bit scorched. Remove. Crack the shell at once with a hammer in several places. The meat inside will have started to pull away from the shell and will be easy to pry loose where it has not loosened already. Pare off the thin brown skin with a sharp paring knife.

If the coconut meat is to be served as a snack, cut into pieces about ½ inch square. If it is to be chopped or shredded, put it on a chopping board and use a long-bladed knife. To shred, put these chunks of coconut meat through a food grinder, using the fine blade.

Dried Shredded Coconut

Remove meat from fresh coconut as described above, put through fine blade of food grinder, then spread out thin in a shallow baking pan and dry in a slow oven (300° F.), stirring occasionally until *completely dry* to the touch. Do not allow to brown. Cool completely, then store in a covered container or in plastic bags.

If coconut is to be given away, when dried put it into thoroughly sterilized small jars with fitted lids. The natural sweetness and full flavor of the coconut are retained; in fact, one wonders why sugar needs to be added to the commercial product.

Cranberry Coconut Relish Mold

2 cups raw cranberries
1½ cups chopped pitted prunes
1 cup coarsely chopped fresh coconut
1 teaspoon grated orange rind

1 envelope unflavored gelatin
¼ cup cold water
1 cup orange juice

Put cranberries through food grinder; drain thoroughly. Add prunes, coconut and orange rind, and stir to blend. Sprinkle gelatin over cold water to soften. Heat orange juice, but do not boil. Add hot juice to gelatin and stir until dissolved. Add mixture of prunes, cranberries, and coconut. Pour into 3-cup mold. Chill until firm. Serve as a relish salad with Thanksgiving dinner or for a buffet. Makes about 10 relish servings.

Note: If a sweeter relish is desired, increase the prunes to 2 cups and use a 3½-cup mold.

To make this into a relish, rather than a gelatin mold, add to the mixture ¼ cup of orange juice and 2 tablespoons of sherry. For a thicker consistency, add 1 tablespoon of honey as well.

Orange Date Chutney

2 large navel oranges	2 cups brown sugar
1 pound pitted dates, chopped	1 tablespoon salt
	1 tablespoon curry powder
3 medium onions	1½ teaspoons cumin seeds
1 garlic clove, minced	½ teaspoon powdered ginger
1 cup seedless raisins	1 cup chopped walnuts
1 quart vinegar	

Carefully peel oranges: remove outer rind so thinly that no white comes with it; cut rind into long, thin strips. Remove all white from fruit and cut fruit in quarters, through the segments. Remove any seeds. Chop oranges and outer peel in blender (or put through food grinder), but save all the juice. Chop the dates, onion, garlic, and raisins into fine pieces, not pureed. If using blender, turn it on, off, on, off repeatedly to prevent the mixture from turning into a paste.

Combine vinegar, sugar, salt, and spices; bring to a boil and boil for 5 minutes. Add orange mixture and walnuts and continue to cook over lowest heat until mixture is reduced and syrup is thickened. Ladle into hot, sterilized jars; cover and twist tight to seal. Store in cool, dry place and use within 2 months. Makes about 3 pints, or 6 half-pints.

Wild Blackberry Sauce

If you spend the summer where there are blackberry bushes growing wild, dress in scratchproof clothing from head to foot, wear garden gloves, and pick as many pails of the berries as you can find. Use some to make a sauce for topping ice cream, the rest for jam.

For the sauce, carefully pick over and wash berries; add 1 cup of sugar to each cup of berries, and place in a large kettle. Bring slowly to a boil; simmer for 5 minutes. Ladle into sterilized jars or jelly glasses, and seal. One quart of berries will make about 3 cups of sauce.

Note: This sauce is not like jam; it must be stored in the refrigerator.

Blackberry Lemon Jam

2 quarts blackberries
9 cups sugar

2 lemons, seeded and finely chopped (with peel)

Wash and pick over berries, removing all hard caps and overripe berries. Place in kettle with sugar and lemons. Let stand for 1 hour; slowly bring to a boil and cook until thickened (about 20 minutes). Ladle into hot, sterilized jars. Cool, then pour melted paraffin over tops and cover with fitted lid. (The paraffin helps to protect the jam but does not prevent spoilage. However, if stored in a cool, dry place, the jam does not require refrigeration and should keep throughout the winter.)

Holiday Fruit Cake

½ cup butter
¾ cup packed dark brown sugar
½ cup unsulfured molasses
3 eggs
1 cup unbleached all-purpose flour
1 cup whole-wheat flour
½ teaspoon soda
¼ teaspoon salt
¼ cup wheat germ

1 teaspoon cinnamon
½ teaspoon allspice
1 teaspoon vanilla
¾ cup peach or apricot nectar
¾ cup chopped pitted dates or prunes
¾ cup currants
¼ cup citron, thinly sliced
¼ cup candied lemon peel
¼ cup chopped nuts
Glacé cherries and citron for garnish

Line 2 loaf pans (9x5x3 inches) with brown paper, then grease paper and dust with flour. Cream together butter and sugar until fluffy. Beat in molasses and eggs until smooth. Combine two flours with soda and salt, stirring to distribute and blend thoroughly. Add wheat germ and spices. Add to butter mixture alternately with fruit nectar; avoid overbeating. Toss fruits and nuts with 2 tablespoons of flour, then stir into the batter, distributing evenly.

Arrange glacé cherries and citron slices in bottom of pans, spoon batter over them, at first using about ½ cup so as not to disturb fruit garnish; then carefully add remaining batter, filling pans almost full. Bake in a slow (300° F.) oven for 2½–3 hours, or until a pick inserted in the center comes out clean and cake has drawn away from the sides of the pan. (If cake browns too quickly during baking, cover top with foil.)

Cool in pans for 10 minutes, then invert on cake racks. When cold, wrap with cheesecloth soaked in brandy, cream sherry, rum, or bourbon. Then wrap in a double thickness of foil or plastic, folding over ends, and store in a cool place to age and mellow. Makes 2 cakes.

(These should be baked at least a month before Christmas so that they can become sufficiently mellow for gift-giving.)

Hutzelbrot
(German Fruit Bread)

3–4 cups unbleached all-purpose flour
½ cup sugar
1 teaspoon salt
1 tablespoon anise or fennel seeds
½ teaspoon ground cinnamon
Pinch of ground cloves
1¾ cups water
⅔ cup finely chopped dried pears
⅔ cup finely chopped dried figs
⅔ cup diced pitted prunes
2 packages active dry yeast
½ cup (1 stick) margarine
3 cups dark rye flour
1 cup chopped toasted almonds
1 cup chopped walnuts
⅓ cup minced candied orange or lemon peel

Place 2 cups of the all-purpose flour in a large mixing bowl. To flour add sugar, salt, anise or fennel seeds, and spices. Place the fruit in another bowl, add 1½ cups of water which has been heated to boiling; let stand for 5 minutes until the fruit softens, then pour off the liquid through a sieve, saving it to use for the bread.

Soften the yeast in ¼ cup of lukewarm water. Make a well in the center of the flour mixture, add the dissolved yeast and the liquid drained from the fruit. Add the margarine (it does not need to be melted) and beat in the flour mixture to make a thick batter. (If using an electric mixer, beat for 2 minutes, scraping down bowl occasionally.) Add the rye flour and more of the unbleached flour, ½ cup at a time, until a soft, pliable dough is formed. Turn out onto lightly floured surface and knead until smooth and elastic. Place in a greased bowl, turning to grease top of dough. Cover with plastic wrap; let rise in warm, protected place until doubled in bulk (about 1 hour).

Punch down dough, turn out again on floured board. Toss nuts, candied peel, and fruit with the remaining flour, then work into the dough as you again knead it, until all the fruit and nuts have been worked in. Divide dough in half; form into 2 round balls. Place on greased baking sheets. Cover lightly; let rise again.

Preheat oven to 375° F. When bread has again doubled, place in oven and bake about 40 minutes, or until crust sounds hollow when tapped. Remove from baking sheets to wire racks. Brush top with margarine for a glossy crust. Do not cut until completely cold. Makes 2 loaves.

Algarve Fig Pastry

FILLING:
¾ cup finely chopped dried figs
½ cup chopped nuts
1 tablespoon light honey
Grated orange or lemon rind
2 tablespoons orange juice

PASTRY:
2 cups unbleached all-purpose flour
⅛ teaspoon salt
¾ cup (12 tablespoons) cold butter
Grated lemon rind
1 egg, beaten
1 tablespoon water
2 tablespoons bran meal (optional)

Prepare filling first: combine ingredients in order given. Set aside. To make pastry: place flour and salt in bowl and mix to blend; then cut in butter until in pieces the size of tiny peas. Add lemon rind, then slowly stir in with a fork the beaten egg mixed with water, tossing mixture until flour is moistened. With fingers, form into a ball, kneading lightly and rolling ball of dough over particles in bottom of bowl so they will adhere to dough. Divide into 2 portions. Press one portion over bottom of 11x7¼x11-inch baking pan (or 9x9-inch pan). Sprinkle bran over the crust, if desired (but with all these figs, it's not really necessary). Spread fig mixture over the crust as evenly as possible. Roll out second portion of dough to fit pan as the top crust. (As this pastry is very short, you may find it easier to pick up the crust after first running a spatula under it.) Place top crust over fig mixture; prick in several places with fork. Bake in preheated hot (400° F.) oven until pastry is golden (about 25 minutes). When cool, cut into squares. Makes 15 squares.

(If this is to be given as a gift, wrap each square separately in plastic wrap.)

Fudgy Oat Brownies

1 package (6 ounces) carob nuggets*
¼ cup butter or margarine
2 eggs
½ cup sugar
1 cup steel-cut or quick-cooking rolled oats
½ teaspoon baking powder
½ teaspoon salt
1 teaspoon vanilla
¾ cup chopped walnuts

Grease an 8-inch-square baking pan. Melt carob nuggets and butter in top of double boiler over hot but not boiling water. In mixing bowl, beat eggs until light, gradually beat in sugar, then stir in oats, baking powder, salt, vanilla, and nuts. When well blended, stir in carob mixture. Spoon into baking pan, spreading evenly. Bake in oven preheated to 350° F. for about 30 minutes, or until top is crisp. Cool. Cut in squares while in pan. Remove from pan when cold, using a spatula. Makes 16.

*If preferred, use chocolate bits instead of carob nuggets.

Easy Coconut Macaroons

2 cups unsweetened shredded coconut
¾ cup sweetened condensed milk

Dash of salt
1 teaspoon vanilla
¼ teaspoon almond extract

Combine ingredients and let stand for 2 or 3 minutes. Preheat oven to 325° F. Spread brown paper over baking sheet and grease the paper. Drop mixture by teaspoonfuls 1 inch apart on paper; flatten with back of spoon. Bake until golden (about 25 minutes). Remove immediately with spatula and cool on a flat surface. Store in covered container. Makes about 3 dozen.

Fruited Macaroons

To above mixture, add ½ cup of chopped pitted dates, or chopped figs or apricots—or a mixture of these fruits. Decrease coconut to 1½ cups.

Hi-Fiber Macaroons

Prepare as in basic recipe but add ¼ cup of whole-bran cereal to mixture.

Coconut Filbert Macaroons

Decrease coconut to 1½ cups, add ½ cup of chopped filberts or hazelnuts (or use slivered brazil nuts).

Honey Nut Squares

¼ cup honey
¼ cup ground dates
¾ cup ground raisins

3 tablespoons wheat germ
1 cup ground nuts

Heat together honey and fruits; stir in wheat germ and nuts and spread out on a shallow greased baking pan. When cold, cut with knife dipped in hot water, to make squares. Makes about 24.

Spiced Pumpkin Cookies

1 egg
½ cup oil
½ cup dark brown sugar
½ cup honey
½ teaspoon vanilla
1 cup canned or cooked
    pumpkin
1¼ cups whole-wheat flour
¼ cup crushed whole-bran
    cereal
1 teaspoon baking soda

½ teaspoon salt
½ teaspoon *each* cinnamon
    and nutmeg
¼ teaspoon powdered ginger
¼ teaspoon crushed
    cardamom
½ cup raisins, chopped
1 cup chopped peanuts
½ cup flaked coconut
Additional coconut for
    garnish

Break egg into mixing bowl, beat until light. Add oil, sugar, honey, and vanilla; stir to blend. Add pumpkin and mix well. Combine dry ingredients, including spices and stir to blend thoroughly. Add flour mixture to pumpkin mixture, ¼ at a time. Stir in raisins, nuts, and coconut. Drop by teaspoonfuls on a lightly greased or Teflon-coated baking sheet. Press down each spoonful with the back of a spoon; place a few shreds of coconut on top of each. (These may be placed fairly close together since they do not spread.) Bake in oven preheated to 375° F. for 15 minutes, or until browned on edges. Makes about 40. Keep stored in covered container.

Fruit Chews

1 cup dried figs
1 cup dried apricots
1 cup pitted dates
½ cup glacé cherries, chopped
1 cup walnut pieces

½ cup shredded coconut
Pinch of salt
2 tablespoons honey
½ cup crushed nuts

Put fruits and walnuts through food grinder; add coconut, salt, and honey to mixture and blend well. Shape into small balls and roll in crushed nuts. Chill. Makes about 4 dozen.

Peanut Carob Chews

2 6-ounce packages carob
   nuggets or swirls
¼ cup milk

½ cup peanut butter
5 cups Wheat Chex crushed
   to 2½ cups

Butter a large bowl and also an 8x8-inch pan. Melt the carob nuggets or swirls in top of double boiler; stir until smooth. Remove from heat. Add milk and peanut butter and stir until thoroughly blended. Put the crushed cereal in the buttered bowl, add the carob-peanut mixture, and stir until cereal is well coated. Press into buttered pan with buttered spoon.

Let stand until cool, then cut into small squares. Remove with spatula and chill. When cold, they can be stored in loosely covered container or wrapped for gift-giving in a waxed-paper-lined box.

Fruit Nut Slices

1½ cups pitted dates
½ cup dried apricots
½ cup chopped dried figs
½ cup unsweetened
   shredded coconut

¼ cup sunflower kernels,
   finely chopped, or crushed
   peanuts
¼ cup wheat germ

Put dates, apricots, and figs through food grinder. Add coconut and sunflower kernels or peanuts. With fingers, press mixture together to form a long roll, about 1½ inches in diameter. Roll in wheat germ. Chill until firm. Cut into slices with sharp floured knife. Keep refrigerated. To give as a gift, separate slices with waxed paper in layers inside a gift box. Makes 12–15 slices.

FOOD COMPOSITION CHARTS

VEGETABLE CHART

Vegetable	% Fiber	Serving Portion	Calories	Fiber in Grams
Artichokes, fresh, whole, cooked	2.4	1 large	8-50	2.8
hearts, frozen or canned	0.9	5-6	24	0.8
Asparagus, fresh or frozen, cooked	0.7	4 spears	14	0.6
Avocado, raw, whole	1.5	½ avocado	185	1.6
diced or sliced	1.2	½ cup	97	1.1
Beet greens, cooked	1.8	½ cup	22	1.2
Beets, cooked or canned, sliced				
or diced	0.8	½ cup	41	0.8
whole	0.8	3 medium	48	1.2
Black-eyed peas, immature,				
fresh or frozen, cooked	1.8	½ cup	88	1.5
Broadbeans (see Italian)				
Broccoli, fresh, cooked	1.6	2 spears	30	2.7
frozen, ⅓ package	1.0	3 small	25	0.95
Brussels sprouts, fresh, cooked	1.6	4 sprouts	56	2.5
frozen, cooked	1.0	⅓ pack.	30	1.04
Cabbage, red, raw	1.0	¾ cup	17	1.1
cooked or canned	1.0	½ cup	62	1.1
Cabbage, white or green, raw	0.8	¾ cup	12	0.9
cooked	0.8	¾ cup	22	0.7
Carrots, fresh, raw	1.0	1 medium	21	0.5
cooked or canned	0.8	½ cup	20	0.8
Cauliflower, fresh, raw	1.0	⅔ cup	19	1.0
fresh or frozen, cooked	0.8	⅓ pack. ⅔ cup	21	0.95
Celeriac (celery root), fresh	1.3	4 ounces	45	1.5
raw or cooked		½ cup	30	0.9
Celery (Pascal), raw	0.7	2 small stalks	9	0.35
cooked	0.7	½ cup	9	0.5
Chard, raw or cooked	0.8	½ cup	17	0.7
Chinese celery or celery cabbage,				
raw or briefly cooked	0.6	½ cup	12	0.5
Collards, fresh, cooked	1.0	½ cup	40	1.2
frozen, chopped	1.1	⅓ pack.	29	1.0
Corn on cob, fresh	0.8	1 small ear	85	0.8

Vegetable	% Fiber	Serving Portion	Calories	Fiber in Grams
Corn, canned kernel	0.8	½ cup	64	0.8
cream style	0.8	½ cup	80	0.8
frozen ears	0.7	1 ear	107	0.98
frozen little ears	0.7	2 ears	70	1.08
Cucumber, with skin	0.6	½ cup	12	0.5
peeled	0.3	½ cup diced	7	0.2
Dandelion greens, raw	1.6	½ cup	44	1.6
cooked	1.3	½ cup	30	1.2
Eggplant, cooked	0.9	½ cup	19	0.9
Endive (Belgian), raw or cooked	0.9	½ cup	20	0.9
or chicory, raw	0.9	¼ pound	23	0.9
Fennel, raw	0.6	¼ pound	23	0.9
Green beans, fresh, raw or cooked	1.0	½ cup	16	0.9
frozen French style	1.2	⅓ pack.	21	1.02
frozen cut	0.9	⅓ pack.	22	0.8
Green peas, fresh, cooked	2.2	½ cup	60	2.0
frozen, cooked	1.9	⅓ pack.	85	1.5
frozen, tiny, cooked	1.7	⅓ pack.	60	1.6
canned, drained	1.7	½ cup	76	1.7
Italian or broadbeans, fresh, immature	1.1	½ cup	30	1.8
frozen, cooked	1.1	⅓ pack.	30	0.9
Kale, fresh, raw	1.3	¼ pound	30	1.1
cooked	1.1	½ cup	15	0.6
frozen, chopped, cooked	1.0	⅓ pack.	29	0.8
Kohlrabi, cooked	1.0	½ cup	18	0.8
Leeks, raw or cooked	1.3	¼ pound	59	1.5
Lettuce, Boston, iceberg	0.5	1 cup	8	0.3
romaine, escarole	0.7	1 cup	8	0.4
Lima beans, fresh, Fordhook (or frozen, cooked)	1.6	½ cup	94	1.5
frozen baby limas	1.8	⅓ pack.	120	1.7
frozen baby butter beans	1.8	⅓ pack.	130	1.7
Mushrooms, fresh, raw	0.8	½ cup	10	0.3
frozen whole, in butter	0.8	⅓ pack.	89	0.3
canned (water pack)	0.8	¼ cup	12	0.35
Mustard greens, fresh, raw or cooked	1.1	½ cup	26	1.0
frozen, chopped, cooked	0.8	⅓ pack.	19	0.76
Okra, fresh, cooked	1.0	½ cup	23	0.9
frozen, whole	0.6	⅓ pack.	35	0.6
frozen, sliced	1.0	½ cup	35	0.9
Olives, green	1.3	6 olives	42	0.6
ripe, Greek style	3.8	1 ounce	96	1.1
ripe, California	1.4	6 olives	36	0.4
Onions, raw or cooked, mature	0.6	¼ cup	20	0.4
green (scallions)	1.0	¼ cup	11	0.25
Parsnips, cooked	2.0	½ cup	50	1.6
Peas and carrots, frozen	1.6	⅓ pack.	46	1.5
Peas and cauliflower (frozen)		⅓ pack.	100	1.4
Peas and celery (frozen)		⅓ pack.	45	1.4
Peppers, green sweet, raw	1.4	¼ cup	8	0.5
green sweet, baked	1.4	1 large	26	1.6
red sweet, raw	1.4	1 ounce	9	1.0
hot red chili, fresh	1.8	½ cup	30	0.9
hot red chili, dried	26.2	½ tsp.	5	0.15

Vegetable	% Fiber	Serving Portion	Calories	Fiber in Gram
Potatoes, white, baked in skin	0.6	1 medium	92	0.6
boiled in skin	0.5	1 medium	92	0.6
mashed	0.4	½ cup	92	0.5
French-fried		10 pieces	156	0.6
raw, pan-fried	1.0	½ cup	101	0.2
dried granules, reconstituted	0.2	½ cup	101	0.2
frozen French fries		10 pieces	125	0.4
potato chips		10 pieces	114	0.3
Pumpkin, cooked or canned	1.3	½ cup	40	1.6
Rutabaga, raw or cooked	1.8	½ cup	30	0.9
Salsify (oyster plant), cooked	1.8	¼ pound	14	2.0
Spinach, raw	0.6	1 cup	14	0.3
cooked	0.6	½ cup	26	1.0
frozen, chopped	0.8	⅓ pack.	26	0.9
Squash, scallop	0.6	½ cup	19	0.7
thin rind yellow	0.6	½ cup	15	0.4
winter squash, baked	1.8	½ cup	56	1.8
winter squash, boiled, mashed		½ cup	39	1.6
winter squash, frozen	1.4	½ cup	46	1.4
zucchini	0.6-0.8	½ cup	20	0.8
Succotash, frozen	0.9	⅓ pack.	80	0.85
Sweet potatoes, baked in skin	0.9	1 large	155	1.0
boiled	0.7	1 large	168	1.0
candied		½ cup	157	0.5
canned, vacuum packed		½ cup	118	1.1
Tomatoes, fresh, raw	0.5	1 medium	33	0.8
cooked or canned	0.6	3 slices	26	0.6
		¾ cup	37	0.8
Turnip, white, raw	0.9	¼ cup	10	0.3
cooked, mashed	0.9	½ cup	26	1.0
Turnip greens, cooked	0.8	½ cup	14	0.5
frozen chopped	0.8	⅓ pack.	22	0.76
Wax beans, *see green beans*				

FRUIT CHART

Fruit	% Fiber	Serving Portion	Calories	Fiber in Grams
Apples, raw, not peeled	1.0	1 apple	80	1.4
raw, peeled	0.6	1 apple	70	0.8
frozen sliced	0.7	⅓ pack.	88	0.65
dried, not cooked	3.1	½ cup	236	2.7
dried, cooked		½ cup	157	1.1
applesauce, canned	0.5	½ cup	116	0.6
Apricots, raw	0.6	2 apricots	32	0.4
canned in syrup	0.4	2 halves	54	0.25
dried, uncooked	3.0	5 halves	50	0.6
dried, cooked		6 halves	99	0.75
apricot nectar		½ cup	68	0.2
Bananas, raw	0.5	1 medium	101	0.6
Blackberries, raw	1.5	½ cup	42	3.0
canned in syrup	2.6	½ cup	125	3.4

Fruit	% Fiber	Serving Portion	Calories	Fiber in Grams
Blueberries, raw	1.5	½ cup	45	1.1
frozen whole	1.5	½ cup	45	1.1
canned in syrup	0.9	½ cup	126	1.1
Boysenberries, *see blackberries*				
Cherries, raw, sour, pitted	0.2	½ cup	45	0.2
raw, sweet, black	0.4	½ cup pitted	57	0.3
canned, water pack	0.1-0.3	½ cup	52	0.1
canned, in syrup	0.3	½ cup	70	0.3
Citron, candied	1.4			
Cranberries, raw	1.4	½ cup	26	0.8
sauce, jellied	0	¼ cup	115	0.15
sauce, whole	0.7	¼ cup	101	0.4
Currants, raw, unsweetened	2.4-3.4	½ cup	27	1.85
Dates, pitted	2.3	3 medium	79	1.5
chopped		¼ cup	119	1.0
Figs, raw	1.2	3 medium	79	1.5
dried, uncooked	5.6	3 medium	190	3.6
canned in syrup	0.7	3 medium	84	0.9
Gooseberries, raw	1.9	½ cup	29	1.4
canned in syrup	1.2	½ cup	50	0.7
Grapefruit, raw	0.2	½	46	0.2
Grapes, raw	0.6	½ cup	30	0.3-0.4
Guavas, raw	5.6	1 average	48	4.4
Kumquats, raw		4 oz.	74	4.2
Lemons, raw, peeled	0.4	½ medium	10	0.15
candied peel	2.3	1 ounce	90	0.7
Loganberries, raw	3.0	½ cup	44	2.15
canned in syrup	1.9	½ cup	40	1.15
Oranges, raw, sliced or diced	0.5	½ cup	53	0.6
Papaya, raw	0.9	½ cup	36	0.8
Peaches, raw	0.9	1 medium	38	0.6
canned in syrup, sliced	0.4	½ cup	32-51	0.5
dried, uncooked	3.1	¼ cup	115	1.4
Pears, raw, unpeeled	1.4	1 pear	101	2.3
raw, peeled	1.0	1 pear		1.9
canned in syrup	0.4	½ cup	87	0.7
dried, uncooked	6.2	—	—	—
dried, cooked	2.6	½ cup	143	3.3
Pineapple, raw	0.4	1 slice	44	0.3
canned unsweetened	0.3	1 slice	90	0.4
chunks frozen	0.3	½ cup	85	0.3
Plums, raw	0.4	2 medium	50	0.5
canned water pack	0.2-0.3	½ cup	70	0.3
canned in syrup	0.3	½ cup	100	0.4
Prunes, uncooked, dried	2.2	½ cup pitted	200	1.2
Raisins	0.9	¼ cup	125	0.4
Raspberries, black raw	5.1	½ cup	25	1.7
red raw	3.0	½ cup	20	1.1
canned black	3.3	½ cup	29	1.9
frozen red, in syrup	2.2	½ cup	122	2.7
Rhubarb, cooked, sweetened	0.6	½ cup	169	0.7
frozen, sweetened	0.8	½ cup	177	1.0
Strawberries, raw	1.3	½ cup	27	1.0
frozen, sweetened	0.8	½ cup	116	0.8
Watermelon, raw	0.3	1 slice	82	1.0

STARCH FOODS
(Side Dishes)

Food	Portion	Calories	Fiber
Bulgur	¾ cup	184	0.9
Chickpeas	¾ cup	180	2.7
Lentils	¾ cup	159	1.8
Macaroni, spaghetti	1 cup	192	0.1
Millet grains	¾ cup	160	1.7
Rice, white, converted	⅔ cup	116	0.1
brown	⅔ cup	135	0.3
instant	⅔ cup	101	0.1
Sweet potato	1 large baked	254	1.6
White beans	¾ cup	177	2.1
White potato	1 large Idaho	139	0.9
	medium, boiled, baked	95	0.7

All above figures are for *cooked* portions.

NUTRITIVE VALUE OF SUGARS
(for Home Use)

Sugar or Sweetener	Portion	Calories	Calcium	Phosphorus	Iron
Brown sugar	1 cup	821	187.0	42	7.5
	½ cup	410	93.5	21	3.75
Honey	½ cup	516	139.5	10	0.85
	1 tbsp.	64	17.0	1	0.1
Molasses, light	½ cup	407	270.0	74	7.0
medium*	½ cup	380	476.0	113	9.5
White sugar	1 cup	770	0	0	0
	1 tbsp.	46	0	0	0

*Commercially, this is labeled "dark molasses." Blackstrap is the third extraction, not listed because it is too bitter to be of use in baking.
None of the above has any fiber whatsoever.

LOW-CALORIE MENUS*

Since most people have pretty much the same breakfast day after day, only general suggestions are given. Lunch at home also seems to be pretty much the same during the week, and those who eat in restaurants must settle for what they can get. Therefore the following are primarily dinner menus.

SUMMER MENUS

Daily Breakfast: Fresh fruit (berries, peaches, bananas)
Easy Granola or whole-grain cereals low in sucrose
Whole-wheat toast or bran muffins
Beverage

Weekend Breakfast: Melon, black cherries, peaches
Scrambled eggs (fiber-enriched)
Muffins
Beverage

Lunches at Home: Cottage cheese mixture, fiber-enriched
Plums, apricots, other fresh fruit
Low-fat milk or tea

Lunches Out: Salad with Oil-Vinegar Dressing
Broiled chicken, fish, sliced ham
Green beans, peas, spinach
Black coffee or tea

Dinner Menus for a Week

Sunday:	Gazpacho with garnishes
	Chicken Barbecue
	Asparagus
	Watermelon
Monday:	Vegetable relishes with Humus Dip
	Stuffed Zucchini
	Fresh green peas with mint
	Egg and Bean Salad
	Jarlsberg cheese, fruit

*Recipes that are capitalized can be found in this book.

Tuesday: Shrimp Apple Dip with yogurt chips
Eggplant Curry with Quick Chutney
Cooked millet
Pachadi (Indian salad)
Melon slice

Wednesday: Senegalese Soup (cold)
Poached Fish with Soybean Parsley Sauce
Dilled carrots
Stir-Fried Sliced Okra
Tomato-cucumber-green bean salad
Sour Rye Caraway Bread (1 slice)
Fresh fruit salad with coconut

Thursday: Tabbouleh (bulgur salad) with lettuce
Broiled steak
Small baked potato
Spinach Catalan
Fresh peaches

Friday: Pickled mushrooms/Stuffed Celery
Hamburgers
Charcoal-broiled Eggplant Kabobs
Corn on cob (1 small)
Salade Algerienne
Blueberries with yogurt

Saturday: Japanese Pork and Vegetable Soup
Moo Goo Gai Pan
Rice or millet
Black cherries for dessert

WINTER MENUS

Daily Breakfasts: Whole orange or half a grapefruit; mixed whole-grain cereal or cooked whole-wheat cereal with low-fat milk; whole-wheat toast with jam (orange marmalade, blackberry, raspberry).

Weekend Breakfast: Strawberries in orange juice, or melon; granola with banana and dried currants; vegetable protein sausages, whole-wheat biscuits.

Lunches at Home: 'Hot vegetable soup, tuna mixture as salad or sandwich, raw apple or pear.

Lunches Out: Hamburger, broiled meat, or sliced lean ham (no bread); salad with Oil-Vinegar Dressing; fruit.

Dinner Menus for a Week

Sunday:	Rye-Flaked Oven-Fried Chicken Escalloped Tomatoes 1 small baked potato Red Cabbage Slaw Orange Date Compote
Monday:	Soybean Supper Soup Quick Bran Loaf Baked Apples (with Raisins)
Tuesday:	Turnip and carrot sticks Swedish Meatballs Potatoes boiled in jackets Pickled Beet Ring Frozen Banana Dessert
Wednesday:	Lamb Stew with Okra Cooked bulgur Winter Salad Red raspberries and sliced bananas
Thursday:	Sweet and Sour Beef Stew Boiled potato Tossed Salad Apple Pineapple Cup
Friday:	Oxtail Soup Carrot Muffins Figs in Orange Juice
Saturday:	Tangy Meatloaf Broccoli Oven-browned Potatoes Canadian Apple Salad (omit nuts) Diced Dried Fruit Compote; or pears with cheese

VEGETARIAN MENUS FOR A WEEK

Assuming that vegetarians, too, stick to much the same breakfast and lunch menus, at least on weekdays, only weekend lunches are suggested.

Sunday:

Lunch:	Grilled cheese on Limpa (rye)
	Coleslaw with apples
	Molasses-sweetened yogurt

Dinner:	Vegetarian-Stuffed Cabbage
	Baked Potatoes
	Caraway Carrots
	Spinach Orange Salad
	Fruit Bowl

Monday Dinner:	Lentil Pottage
	Eggplant and Green Pepper
	Greek Salad with Feta Cheese
	Carrot Cake

Tuesday Dinner:	Succotash Chowder
	Parsnips
	Whole-Wheat Dinner Rolls
	Tossed Salad
	Apple Bran Betty

Wednesday Dinner:	Vegetarian Chow Mein
	Fried Brown Rice
	Canned apricots with coconut
	Cheese and Triscuits

Thursday Dinner:	Baked Stuffed Vegetarian Peppers
	Garbanzos with Yams
	Artichoke hearts salad
	Red Raspberry Slump

Friday Dinner:	Baked Stuffed Tomatoes
	Peas and carrots
	Broccoli or brussels sprouts
	Orange and Avocado Salad
	Raspberry Parfait

Saturday:
  Lunch: Curried Dahl with Egg Wedges
                   Tossed salad with apple and raw
                       mushrooms
                   Herb tea

  Dinner: Fruit Cup
                   Boston Baked Beans (with vegetable-
                       protein sausages)
                   Fruited Boston Brown Bread
                   Spinach Salad
                   Torta di Ricotta

Bibliography

Brody, Jane, "Daily Diet Is Key Factor in Cancer, Studies Show," New York Times News Service, December, 1975.

Burkitt, Denis, interview with, "Our Threshold of Health" (staff written), *Saturday Evening Post,* September, 1975.

Burkitt, Denis, and Painter, N.S., "Dietary Fiber and Disease," *JAMA,* August 19, 1974.

Church, Charles Frederick, and Church, Helen Nichols, "Food Values of Portions Commonly Used," Philadelphia, J.B. Lippincott, 1975.

Cleave, T.L., *The Saccharine Disease.* New Canaan, Conn.: Keats Publishing, 1975.

Cooper, Lenna; Barber, Edith; Mitchell, Helen; Rynbergen, Henderika, *Nutrition in Health and Disease.* Philadelphia: J.B. Lippincott, 1958.

Dairy Council Digest, "The Role of Fiber in the Diet," Vol. 46, No. 1, January-February, 1975.

Danhof, Ivan, "Dietary Fiber: Fad, Fact, Fiction?" paper read before American Dietetic Association, October, 1975.

Dufty, William, *Sugar Blues.* Radnor, Penna.: Chilton Publishing Co., 1975.

Fredericks, Carleton, *The High Fiber Way to Total Health.* New York: Pocket Books, 1976.

Hewitt, Jean, *The New York Times Natural Foods Cook Book.* New York: Avon Books, 1972.

Kraus, Barbara, *The Barbara Kraus Guide to Fiber in Foods.* New York: New American Library, 1975.

Lappé, Frances Moore, *Diet for a Small Planet.* New York: Ballantine Books, 1975.

Mayer, Jean, Professor of Nutrition, Harvard University, several of his syndicated columns, New York Daily News Syndicate.

McCoy, Clive M., "A Nutrition Authority Discusses Mrs. E. G. White," three articles reprinted from Seventh Day Adventist publication, *Review and Herald,* February, 1959.

Morris, Bailey, "Food Additives," two-part series, Washington *Star,* November 28 and 29, 1975.

Pekkanen, John, and Falco, Mathea, "American Sweet Tooth; Its Bitter Aftermath," two-part series, Washington *Post,* June, 1975.

Phillips, Roland, "Cancer in Seventh Day Adventists: Implications for the Role of Nutrition in Cancer," *Cancer Research Journal,* November, 1975, supplement.

Reuben, David, *The Save Your Life Diet.* New York: Random House, 1975.

Rossiter, Al, Jr., "Cholesterol Fact and Fantasy: Is the Egg a Villain?" UPI release, January 15, 1976.

Siegal, Sanford, *Dr. Siegal's Natural Fiber Permanent Weight Loss Diet.* New York: Dial Press, 1975.

USDA Handbook No. 8, *Composition of Foods.*

White, Ellen Gould, *The Ministry of Healing,* and *Medical Science and the Spirit of Prophecy.* Loma Linda, California: Pacific Press.

Index